SCREWING THE RULES

THE NO-GAMES GUIDE TO LOVE

LAUREL HOUSE

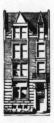

RUNNING PRESS
PHILADELPHIA · LONDON

Published by Running Press,
A Member of the Perseus Books Group

Books published by Running Press are available at special discounts for bulk purchases in the United States by corporations, institutions, and other organizations. For more information, please contact the Special Markets Department at the Perseus Books Group, 2300 Chestnut Street, Suite 200, Philadelphia, PA 19103, or call (800) 810-4145, ext. 5000, or e-mail special.markets@perseusbooks.com.

ISBN 978-0-7624-5408-2
Library of Congress Control Number: 2014946604
E-book ISBN 978-0-7624-5535-5

9   8   7   6   5   4   3   2   1
Digit on the right indicates the number of this printing

Edited by Cindy De La Hoz
Designed by Joshua McDonnell
Typography: Avenir, Garamond, and Lato

Running Press Book Publishers
2300 Chestnut Street
Philadelphia, PA 19103–4371

Visit us on the web!
www.runningpress.com

Contents

INTRODUCTION 7

Here I Am   12

The So-Called Rules and How They Played a Role in
My Failed Relationships   15

CHAPTER 1: ADDRESSING YOUR ISSUES 18

Would You Date Yourself?   19

Love You … First   20

Embracing Your Baggage   23

Get Unstuck from Old Pain: U Dig Strategy   24

Silencing That Broken Record in Your Head   40

CHAPTER 2: WHAT DO YOU NEED? 47

Stop Looking for What You Want and Get What You Need   48

Screw Tall, Dark, and Handsome (Why Looks Don't Matter
When It Comes to True Love)   52

Love May Be Blind, but Chemistry Is Blinding   56

How to Be Attracted to the Right Guy for You   58

Love On-Purpose   61

Define Your Core Values   63

Purpose + Core Values = Your Best Self   67

Intention Board: How Do You Want to Feel?   71

Get a Life Before You Get a Boyfriend   73

Get Real! First Date Conversations: Framing Your Stories   75

CHAPTER 3: HOW TO GET HIM 83

Must-Have Feminine Traits to Catch and Keep a Great Man 84

X Appeal: The Alluring, Captivating, and Intoxicating Trait
That Most Women Lack 89

How to Walk into a Room and Own It 90

How to Flirt 93

Feminine Communication: Phone, E-mail, Text: The Dos,
Don'ts, and What to Expect 107

Icebreakers and Conversation Starters 115

Simple but Stressed-Over First-Date Basics 123

How to Be an Expert Online Dater 130

Essential Prequalifying Strategy to Never Have a
Bad First Online Date Again 138

Prequalifying Questions to Vet Him Before Giving *Any*
Personal Info 143

Love Is a Skyscraper: Go Down Before You Go Up 147

Talk About Your Ex 153

Friend Zone and Booty Calls: How to Avoid Them 159

If You're Not Interested, He's Crazy About You—
If You *Are*, He's Not 168

Attitude of Abundance 169

The Make or Break: Vacation Date 170

CHAPTER 4: HOW TO KEEP
HIM . . . AND SEX 172

The Danger of Having Such Power Over Men 172

Wedding Cake Love 173

When Should You Have Sex? 178

There Are Also Dangers of *Waiting* to Have Sex 182

"I Hate My Body" . . . Is Ruining Your Sex Life 184

How to Be the Best He's Ever Had . . . in Bed 186

CHAPTER 5: LOVE AND (EVENTUALLY ... MAYBE) MARRIAGE 189

Should You Give Your Man an Ultimatum? 189

What Is He Waiting For? 191

What's the Rush? 192

Flirting, Lingerie, and Oral Sex: Put Some Effort into Your Relationship! 194

Monthly Check-Ins 199

Nightly Thank-Yous 200

CHAPTER 6: WHEN TO CALL IT QUITS AND GET OVER HIM 202

I Miss Your Smile, but I Miss Mine More: When to End It 202

How to Break Up 204

Now What? 210

When You Have No Choice but to Break Your Own Heart 212

Eight Steps to Stop Obsessing Over Him 214

Unhooking: Ending a Toxic Relationship with an Ex 216

CHAPTER 7: YOU CAN HAVE IT ALL 220

ACKNOWLEDGMENTS 223

The information in this book is powerful. I am revealing the secret strategy to get a guy to fall in love with you—deep, hard, and fast. And I don't mean that in a sexual way (though it can also lead to having the best sex of your life). Once you learn how to harness this power over men, it's up to you to wield it responsibly.

But to obtain this power, you're going to have to be open to the process—which you must be because you picked up this book. You have finally come to the realization that what you have been doing hasn't been working. You are tired of the games, the runaround, the wondering what you did wrong, the relationship rut, the insecurities, the confusion, the miscommunication . . . And you're ready to find love. Just know that to get it (which you will!), you're going to have to work for it. I will challenge you to get out of your comfort zone and try things that might make you feel awkward or stupid, and I will walk you into some deep and painful crevices of yourself—areas that you shut down and made off-limits long ago.

What I am teaching you is a skill. As with any skill, practice is essential in the process of mastery. You will make mistakes, you may be triggered or relapse into old habits, and you might even hurt others or yourself along the way. Just remember that it's not how many times you fall; it's how many times you get back up that matters.

Not to worry, the painful stuff in this process is mostly at the beginning. This is going to be fun—*yes*, dating can be a blast! But finding love is even better. If you're ready (and I know you are), let's get started.

Dating isn't about games. It's about strategy.
What's the difference?
Games are for fun and manipulation.
Strategy is about dating smart and on-purpose.
So SCREW the "Rules" that dictate the games.
It's time to date strategically and on-purpose.

Introduction

- Do you wonder, "How is it that *she* is in a relationship and I'm not?"
- Do you have difficulty being feminine because you fear appearing weak and powerless?
- Do you wonder what you're doing wrong and why you can't get a second date?
- Do you consistently get questioned, "How are you *still* single? You're such a catch!"
- Do you look at other smiling couples and wish you could feel that loved too?
- Do you wake up next to your boyfriend/fiancé/husband and think, "Is this it?"
- Do you feel lonelier when you're with him than you do when you're alone?
- Honestly . . . do you still fantasize about your first love?

And after those insecurities run through your mind, do you automatically erect your comforting walls that reassure you that there are no good guys in your city; all of the guys you meet are either idiots, assholes, players, or taken; guys are just too intimidated by your success, strength, beauty, etc.

Are any of those reasons really true, or could there be other influences at play? Maybe a deep-seated insecurity that is blocking you from dropping the walls and allowing someone in?

It's so easy to blame your location, men in general, or other factors for your inability to get and keep a good guy. I'm absolutely not declaring that you are at fault either . . . Though you may be. Most likely, the issue isn't you or him. It's your strategy. It's those rules, that list, your set of prerequisites that have been leading you astray. Well, screw them! There are a lot of great, single, dedicated, faithful, totally-your-type, good guys in your town who are looking for a fab chick exactly like you. It's time to find, attract, grab, and keep him instead of letting some other woman nab him up while you're looking the other way.

Screwing the Rules is the no-games way to find the right guy at the right time—right now. Start by becoming your best self (which we will work on together) so you can attract equally awesome guys, have the strength and confidence to show weakness and vulnerability, form a deeply rooted connection and firm foundation, then build a fabulous and fulfilling relationship—one that lasts this time. How? By being smart, getting raw, and having a strategy. And that's what I reveal.

Some of the long-trusted dating books from yester-decades are criticized by readers for encouraging dishonesty, distance, and manipulation. Though claiming not to be about playing games, many of these relationship guides are veritable playbooks on how to be a Stepford wife, from initial hook to coyly reeling him in without ever revealing too much about yourself, instead presenting the perfect virginal woman. The most well known of these rule books is *The Rules,* which states in the introduction that its guidelines are indeed old-fashioned, passed down from generation to generation—literally great-grandma's rules from "circa 1917." The problem with that is that gender roles, and therefore dating and relationship engagement, were simple a hundred years ago. Women weren't CEOs. We weren't earning the bread; we were baking it. We were nurturers, caregivers, moms, and wives, and we are still all of those things . . . And so much more. While, sure, some of us still want the stay-at-home lifestyle (which is fine and dandy too!), we now have the option to choose.

Fact is, we as a society and as individuals have changed. We are shaking up the conventional system of marrying young, having kids, building our careers, and living happily ever after (or at least sticking together, happily or not). We are fast paced and moving full speed ahead, but simultaneously we are taking longer to wed and having children in all sorts of unconventional ways. Yeah, definitely not the same chick from the dependent '20s, stay-at-home '50s, or even swinging '70s. We are putting our careers first and focusing on love and kids later. The result: life experience. We are seeing and doing more. We are becoming more opinionated and sure of our wants. We have higher expectations, bigger dreams, and more focused fantasies. We are also becoming more rigid, less romantic, and less tolerant of BS. We have fortified our hearts with protective walls, the residual of old fears, pain, and baggage. We are creating lists and requirements that must be met in order to move forward. We have become used to having an opinion that matters, making demands, and putting ourselves first.

All of that said, we still want the one thing that most women have always craved, no matter what decade or headspace we're in: love. If we want timeless desires to be fulfilled, we need to tweak the conventional dating rules that no longer apply and retool them for today. It is absolutely possible and acceptable to be simultaneously strong and vulnerable, opinionated and submissive, focused and free, controlling and cared for, hardworking and easygoing, even traditional and independent. You are a strong, sexy, feminine woman—an independent traditionalist. Embrace it!

And what about those games? Hate them, don't you? Well, guess what? Most of the games you play are rooted in those conventional rules—dating expectations that dictate when you should call or not call, make yourself available or pretend to be busy, and tip-toe around the truth—which isn't lying; it's just not being exactly transparent. Well, screw the rules! It's time to get real. The no-games approach will help you break down your barriers, be your authentic self, and create a strategy to finally meet Mr. Right-for-You.

It's time to be honest about who you are and what makes you happy, embody your best self, be raw with your emotions, show your weak side sometimes, and embrace who you are—baggage and all. Once we've got you figured out and dateable, I will teach you the formula to attract the right guy for you and to get what for a lot of you is the end goal: your guy kneeling down—on the solid foundation that you two built—and putting a ring on your finger.

This book is different from all of the other dating books you have read. Unlike some relationship coaches, I'm not a therapist who learned about love and its various complications and incarnations from textbooks. These techniques also haven't been passed down from my great-grandma. I'm a dating expert with real and extensive experience in the field. I have made enough mistakes for a busload of women. I followed the rules and got what I thought I wanted, disappointed myself and my family, and acted carelessly and recklessly (with myself and others). I fell for bad boys who hurt me in an array of ways. I failed to meet my expectations. I had my heart shredded and became a rigid bitch out of fear of opening up again. I got the third degree from myself (my biggest and harshest critic). I analyzed and broke down my breakups and extracted the lessons; I excavated and aired my baggage, endured, and then learned from countless hours of therapy. In the process I developed a strategy to attract great guys, make them want to commit, and get them to fall in love ... quickly. And I *experienced, experienced, experienced* to the tune of two marriages, three engagements, and nine proposals (more on that later).

I have truly been there and done pretty much all of it, and I have the stories, perspective, and insight to help make your trek less treacherous. This isn't a mild-mannered book filled with esoteric ideals on emotional surrender and spiritual depth. This is a practical guide that will actually spell out exactly what to do to become your best self, get the guy you want and deserve, and keep him. It's filled with real advice plus examples of lots of my own mistakes. Don't expect sugarcoating. I'm going to give it to you straight, challenge you to get out of your box and do things differently this time so that you finally find *the* one, not just another *some*one.

Some of my advice is unconventional. It may even be uncomfortable at first—but it works. Now, you may be saying, you don't want to "change" yourself to attract the right guy. You want to let love come "naturally." You believe that your right guy will appear at the right time. You can't force love. You don't want to seem like you're trying too hard or desperate, so you'd rather just keep doing what you're doing because it's "easier."

You're right about a few things:

You shouldn't have to change for a guy. But you *can* work on becoming your best self first—physically and emotionally. You can expand your interests so that you become more interesting (it's tough to keep a guy interested if you're uninteresting). You can come to love yourself so much that you radiate confidence from the inside out (the most attractive trait that draws men in!). Then you will have the ability to attract an equally incredible man.

You can't force love. But you can put yourself in the right place at the right time to attract chemistry.

You don't want to appear desperate or like you're trying too hard. But it goes way beyond not "appearing" desperate: you don't want to *be* desperate, and you won't be when you're attracting so many amazing men. And you certainly won't be "trying" too hard, because you will be completely comfortable about just being you.

It's easier to keep doing what you're doing. But how do you feel at night when you go to bed alone or when you go to bed with the wrong guy . . . again? Don't you deserve more and better? I'll answer that for you. You *do* deserve much more and much better. You deserve to be happy.

Strategy takes effort. But so does anything that's worthwhile, right? Think about your career. Did you just sit there and wait for a company to come knock on your door and offer you your dream job? Or did you work your ass off to build your resume, expand your experience, perfect your abilities, make yourself into the best candidate for the position, put yourself in the right place at the right time, then sell yourself so that your potential boss or client would see just how awesome you are?

To be honest, I'm a little nervous right now. I am putting myself out on a platter (or more accurately, in a book) for you to consume—flaws and all. Some of the stories that I am about to reveal are me at my worst and weakest. But here I am. I don't believe that you are judging me. If you don't like me, that's okay. Maybe we aren't a fit. But I like me. And I'm not judging you either. In fact, it's an attitude of "Here I am" that I hope you are able to adopt from this book. It's a simple attitude adjustment. That's it! Here I am. No judgment.

Not sure what I mean? What if, when you walk into a party, meet your date, or even enter a meeting, you think, "Here I am," instead of, "Here I am, what do you think?" or "Here I am, do you like me?" or "Here I am, am I good enough for you?"

Many of us have the expectation of judgment. We immediately give our power away, lowering ourselves to assume the worst. Here's the problem—well, there are many problems with this situation, but one of the biggies is that we are putting our own critical self-judgment on others. And they can feel it. And what happens when they feel it? They believe it too. You are essentially saying, "Here, let me give you these dirty, tainted glasses that I see myself through, so that you can see me the way I do."

Another problem is that as soon as you start thinking it, you'll start acting it. Think it, act it, be it—right? Think, "I'm not good enough," "I'm not smart enough," "He can do better than . . ." and guess what? You'll act that way. You'll make your own bed and then you'll have to sleep in it.

It's such a simple shift, but it can change your attitude, your relationships, and your life.

So . . . here I am.

PROFESSIONALLY . . .

I am an international dating and relationship coach, flirting and femininity expert, and MTV's *MADE* "It Girl" dating and confidence-boosting mentor. For the last fifteen years I have been writing about everything from sex to fitness, beauty to travel, as an expert and insider. But what I love to write about the most is sex and dating. I gained invaluable insight on how the male mind works, what it needs versus what it wants, while writing for *Playboy, Men's Journal, Men's Health,* and *FHM.* With more than 15 million views on YouTube, I was voted one of the top ten dating vloggers on the Internet, and I have dating columns on several dating and general lifestyle websites. In all my work, my hope is to use what I've learned to inform, inspire, and empower women who may not have the know-how or experience; are on the wrong path or looking for the wrong guy; or lack the confidence or the awareness of how they are portraying themselves to put their best selves out there; but desperately want love.

PERSONALLY...

I have had my heart broken, and I have broken my own heart, as well as the hearts of others. I have lived and loved and learned ... a lot!

I am a risk taker when it comes to love. I tear open my chest to expose my heart, travel to the other side of the world, take a leap instead of a step, and put my entire self into my relationships. Sometimes I fall, fail, and make a fool of myself. Sometimes I get hurt and end up curled in a tear-soaked ball on the floor. Sometimes I crash and burn, and other times I simply lose steam, but I always emerge more educated and with an expanded understanding of myself and others. And, best of all, sometimes I get to tap into the deepest, most guttural and ecstatic emotions that electrify my existence and remind me why, no matter how much pain it can give us, we can't help ourselves but to crave and do just about anything for love.

I've been described as "like one of the guys" in terms of how I think, but still completely feminine. I have also been called a "man whisperer" for my ability to get in a man's mind and get out what I want. I have been criticized and praised for my abilities. It's the criticism that (no matter how mean) I put to constructive use in order to improve myself and my techniques.

Some people may think my methods are crazy. But somehow my rule screwing has worked, at least when it comes to getting great guys to fall

In love with me and even propose. As I said earlier, I have been married twice, engaged a third time, and proposed to a total of nine times. Almost every first date has led to being asked on a second (except maybe two). "I love you" has been uttered to me a couple dozen times, and "you're wife material" almost as often. I'm not saying any of this to show off, come across as a bitch, or say that I'm in any way more awesome than anyone else. I'm not by any means model-beautiful, I don't have a perfect body, I have lots of baggage, I can be a pain in the ass, and I am most certainly flawed in many ways. I am über-feminine and flirty yet still strong and deliberate. I am quirky yet confident. I'm myself and I own it.

THE SO-CALLED RULES AND HOW THEY PLAYED A ROLE IN MY FAILED RELATIONSHIPS

Although I have never been a strict rule follower, I used to follow some conventional dating rules, and not only didn't they serve me, but they hurt me and in the end hurt others, too. The values behind these rules made me seem careless with others' hearts, beliefs that contributed to my getting divorced—twice.

MY FIRST MARRIAGE WAS TO MY COLLEGE SWEETHEART

We were, quite simply, too young. We married two weeks after graduation and two weeks before my first day at a very competitive shark tank of a company and industry. I changed dramatically and almost immediately. Some couples who marry young luck out, changing and growing together. Others are stunted by their relationships, as the confines of the marriage restrict them from fully stretching their wings and exploring the edges of their being—and that's okay with them. And then there are the individuals who grow, expand, and explore themselves and their potential, then look back to see that their partner didn't grow at the same speed, didn't expand to the same spot, or may have simply taken a divergent path, an opposing fork in the road—and then what? You either decide to accept your differences and remain together or you begin to find that those differences didn't just create distance but tension, friction, and losing touch . . . leading to a separation. And that's what happened to my first marriage. Plus, I pretty much allowed my work to become my priority and take over my life, as I watched myself transform into a bitch.

MY SECOND HUSBAND PROPOSED
WITHIN THREE MONTHS

That pretty much fit the traditional dating rules goal of marriage, in the shortest time possible, to a man you love, who loves you even more than you love him. Three months was fast. But it was particularly fast considering that, although we did "know" each other, we didn't know each other with much emotional depth before he popped the question. As dictated by those rules, I held my cards close to my chest and didn't show all sides of me. I wasn't raw or completely real. I played the games—the games that help you maintain control without letting your guard down, games that don't let you open up or get too close too fast. We got engaged, he started a new, extremely demanding career, and I dove into wedding-planning mode—neither of which were exactly conducive to getting to know each other much better. Within less than a year of meeting, we were married, and then we started to get to know each other and get to know that we were very different from each other. We tried for a couple of years, but we simply were not compatible and we were not happy.

YEARS LATER I GOT ENGAGED A THIRD TIME

I really wanted it to work, but we were unhealthy on multiple levels. Thankfully, I learned from my first two that I needed more in a marriage. I needed deeper. I needed real and raw and honest. I needed our core values to align. I needed to be better and stronger as a couple than I was as an individual. And although a lot of our relationship was great, we, I, and it still needed work. We were not ready for matrimony, and I wasn't going to be that fool who again rushed in.

Translation: I live and work . . . dating. Let my failures help fortify you, point out the pitfalls, help navigate the moments of insecurity, and basically help you avoid the same mistakes I made (because I have made enough for everyone).

You are a castle. You have an edifice that is protected by a wall. That wall is your façade. It may be defensive or beautiful, passive or "perfect," or a combination of all four and more. But what that wall is really doing is hiding you. It's not letting your authentic side, your vulnerable side, your *real* side be revealed, exposed—hurt. Behind that wall is the building. It's YOU. But, instead of a castle, too many women have this little shit house made up of all of their shame, insecurities, baggage, and, well, all that shit that they collected and piled on throughout their life. Or it may be a weak, flimsy, house of cards that can hardly stand on its own because, like a muscle, it has atrophied from lack of use, depending completely on the strength of the protective wall—its crutch..

My first goal in this book is to build up that little house into a castle, so that you no longer need that wall to hide behind and you are a complete and strong woman on your own. Once your castle is built, then you can pretty it up with X Appeal and flirting skills so that you attract an equally amazing, whole, complete man who complements your strengths, fills in your weaknesses, and treats you like the queen that you are, just as you treat him like he is your king. Mutual adoration, respect, love, and the feeling that I am so lucky are the goals. I will help you get there.

Love . . . from the inside out.

CHAPTER 1

Addressing Your Issues

I was a bad wife when I was first married. Sure, I was way too young, completely inexperienced, had no idea who I was or what I stood for (despite being extremely driven and strident), and was in no way ready to be married. It's not that I cheated, indulged in addictions, or partied hard. I was just . . . A miserable bitch. I was controlling and demanding, demeaning, never satisfied, selfish, nagging, and cold. I refused to let my guard down, be vulnerable and soft, or put in any effort. Outsiders didn't see it, though. I worked hard at painting a picture of wedded perfection, replete with a tall, dark, and seriously handsome husband, white picket fence around our adorable red-doored house, and a 130-pound dog named Ruby.

Here's the thing though—I loved *being* a wife. I loved working side by side as we tended to our garden, using our hand-nurtured produce to toss together healthy and delicious meals each night, and sitting on the sofa watching the news at the end of each evening before getting into bed drifting off to sleep.

But although I loved the role, I wasn't being real. I really wanted to fit squarely into the "good wife" mold. We lived the quintessential life and had a perfectly cookie-cut home on the type of street that might appear in a surreal Jim Carrey movie where each home has a manicured lawn and the neighbors smile and wave with that beauty queen pose and give you an "everything's just peachy" grin as you pass by. Mature oak trees and purple flowering jacarandas dotted the sidewalks. It screamed potluck dinners and oozed family. That's why we picked it. But that wasn't me. Not back then at least. I still had a lot of growing to do.

WOULD YOU DATE YOURSELF?

- Would you date you if you were him?
- Would you date someone who has your issues?

Think about your insecurities, your manic behaviors, your internal monologue that tells you how fat and stupid and ugly you are, your criticism of yourself and others, your lies, your dirty laundry, your unfinished business, your self-sabotaging behaviors, your secrets, your MO, your superficiality, your depthless conversations, your workaholic obsession, your inflated or deflated ego, your addictions, your lack of friends, your dysfunctional relationship with your family, your attitude and actions. Would you date someone like that? Would you date you?

If you just read the above and thought, "I'm not so bad, actually. Yes, I would totally date me. In fact, I think I'm a pretty great catch!" then you're either delusional, lying to yourself (and what's the point of that—really?), or you're totally right—you're awesome! Regardless, there are likely areas that can use some improvement (or a total overhaul). So keep reading and get ready to become your best self so that you can attract an incredible guy who complements what you put out and is ready to dive in.

Are you happy? This has nothing to do with anyone else but you. It's not about whether you're in a happy relationship or whether you're having a good or a bad day. Are you happy with yourself? Do you like you? Do you enjoy spending time with you? Or are you easily bored when you're alone? Do you feel like you need the company of other people to enjoy yourself? Or maybe you like to torture yourself by sitting alone and steeping in misery.

For you to be in a happy, healthy, and loving relationship, you need to first be happy, healthy, and in love with yourself.

It's said that people who get bored easily are boring. Same goes for love. If you don't love you, why would he? In the next chapter I'm going to ask you to do some work—writing down your core values, framing your stories, creating an intention board, and determining your purpose. These exercises are all intended to help you get to know yourself a bit better and realize just how amazing, confident, and interesting you really are. But truly, at the very core of all of this, at the core of dating and attracting a great guy and having a happy, healthy, and fulfilled relationship with an amazing partner who supports, complements, and loves you, is a love of yourself. You need to know that you deserve the most incredible guy, who treats you well, respects who you are, and encourages you to continue to grow and be your best self. But you will only attract that person if you truly do believe that you deserve it. If you don't feel that you are worthy, good enough, or deserving of such greatness because you yourself question whether you truly are great, you'll be hard pressed to find someone else who does. Why? Because you won't let yourself. You will only allow yourself to be loved as much as you love yourself.

If you continue to attract guys who treat you like shit; are demeaning, dismissive, abusive; who don't show up, don't follow through, or don't support you, stop wondering what's wrong with all of these assholes and instead see them as a reflection of something within you.

What does your inner voice tell you? How does it speak to you? Does it shut you down or build you up? Would you say the nasty things that you say to yourself to your best friend? Or your worst enemy? Stop being your worst enemy. Change the voice in your head. When you start to hear horrible things being said, literally say, "Enough, that's not true." Why continue to lie to yourself? Are you truly stupid? Really? You're stupid? You're uneducated? Are you honestly hideously ugly? Is your body repulsive? Really? Or is that just a lie too? Would it stand up in court? If someone said that to your best friend, would you defend your friend or let that person continue to trash-talk her? Stop lying to yourself. Stop being your worst enemy. Your words become your reality. The more you bash yourself, your worth, your life, the worse it will be and the more miserable you will become. Let me tell you right now—THAT is not attractive to anyone, and it's certainly not a way to get a great guy.

It's time to start doing things that make you happy. Pamper yourself. Take time for yourself. Explore secret passions. Go on a solo retreat that forces you to refocus on yourself and strengthen the bond that you have with you. If you want a guy to treat you like a treasure, you have to set the standard and treat yourself that way first. Date yourself! Whatever you want a man to do for you, do for yourself. Why? (1) So you can get used to how it feels to be treated that way! (2) To set the precedent. If he sees how well you treat yourself, he will elevate his expectation of himself, knowing that he has to raise the stakes. Why would you be with him if he can't make your life better in some way? What does he have to offer to you that you can't provide for yourself? That doesn't mean that he has to have and spend a lot of money on pampering you. He can cook you dinner, bring you one flower, give you a long massage, take you on an architecture tour of your city. Whatever it is, he is rising to the occasion to prove his worth to you. As he should!

FIRST ASSIGNMENT: DATE YOURSELF

Do one thing every single day that is totally selfish and makes you completely happy. Need a few ideas? Take a bubble bath, sign up for a cooking class, go on a hike, get lost in your favorite erotica audio book, buy yourself a bouquet of your favorite scented flowers, pick up a travel guide for your city and start going on field trips as if you were a tourist, or give yourself some loving . . . yeah, *that* kind. You want to go into your next relationship as a happy, emotionally healthy, and whole person—not a half person looking for happiness from someone else. "You complete me" is sweet, but it's horseshit. You balance me—now *that's* what the goal is! You complete you. He completes him. You are each individually amazing. But you are even more awesome together! Love you . . . first. And soon you will attract someone else to love you, too.

SECOND ASSIGNMENT: I LOVE ME, FIVE WAYS A DAY

Every morning, before you get out of bed or even open your eyes, I want you to think of five things that you love about yourself. Two of those things must be physical. When you get out of bed, immediately write them in a journal. This will be your "I Love Me: Five Ways a Day" journal.

Not into journaling? Not a problem. Write love notes to yourself on Post-its and place them around your house, in your car, or on your computer. Take a dry-erase pen and write your five ways that you love you on your bathroom mirror. Write them on a notecard and stick it in your purse. The point is to think it, say it, and write it…and soon you will truly come to believe it.

Why can't you find the perfect man? Because the perfect man doesn't exist. And by the way, you're not perfect either. But you know that. So stop being so hard on yourself.

It's time to shift the way you view your baggage. So maybe you're divorced, struggled with addictions, came from a broken home, went through a tough or toxic period, dated a little too prolifically, experienced abuse, were imprisoned, hurt yourself or others, acted carelessly, etc., etc. So what? The point isn't the act; it is how you have acted since then. What have you learned? How have you grown? Are you better, stronger, wiser, more evolved, introspective, aware, tender, empathetic, or resilient because of it?

Don't let your baggage weigh you down. Use it to bolster yourself. Stop hating, pitying, or hiding yourself—that's your own form of emotional abuse. Sure, you may have fucked up—maybe big time. But you are who you are today because of your experiences in the past. By saturating in, running from, or covering up those past hardships, you are keeping yourself tethered to them. You are defining yourself by them. You are punishing yourself for them. You aren't allowing yourself to be wholly present or to move forward into a healthy and happy future. Forgive yourself. What you did or what was done to you isn't who you are. We all make mistakes and have shitty experiences. Once you allow yourself to extract the positives from the pain in the form of lessons, then learn from them and change because of them, you can move on and up.

And here's the interesting thing: the harder, more judgmental, and less forgiving you are on yourself, the harder, more judgmental, and less forgiving you are on others. By embracing your baggage and forgiving yourself for your past, you admit that you aren't perfect. No one is. And that "ideal" guy for you? He's imperfect too.

I am about to get very vulnerable with you. This is hard for me. I am doing it because I want you to see the real me. Not the "me" that is out there for public consumption. I want you to see my struggles and know that you are not alone in yours. I hope that in my sharing this with you, you will feel comfortable to open yourself up, too.

I am going to do what I call a U Dig Strategy (which you will learn about after my story). This "U" is intended to excavate and move away from limiting beliefs that keep you stuck in patterns and habits that don't allow you to have the type of healthy and loving relationship that you deserve.

This is the headspace that I was in not too long ago.

LIMITING BELIEF: I'M NOT GOOD ENOUGH

Write down what your life would look like

if you let go of this limiting belief.

If I was able to let go of this limiting belief of feeling like I'm not good enough, I would be able to be in a real and deep relationship with a man who loves me for me and who I love for him.

If I was able to let go of this limiting belief, I would be able to get married—for good this time—and start the family that I so desperately want to have.

If I was able to let go of this limiting belief, I would stop hurting other people in an attempt to protect myself and I would be able to forgive myself for hurting people in the past.

Write down where this belief came from and the events in your life

that reinforced the belief, cementing it into your mind as "truth."

This belief started unknowingly when I was a very little girl. My parents were young, just starting in their careers, and both worked full-time. So they did the absolute best they could afford to do at the time, which was leave me during the day with a woman whose job it was to make sure I didn't die. But she didn't hold me or love me. That wasn't her job. Realizing that I needed to be cared for by someone who cared, my parents found a nanny for me, who turned out to also have a side job as a hooker. Of course, they had no idea about that side job until she was arrested. Then they found an amazing woman who moved in with my family and took incredible care of us—me and my younger siblings when they were born. But the seed was already planted. *I wasn't good enough for love.*

This limiting belief of not being good enough was reinforced when I was in middle school. A very late bloomer, I was unattractive and awkward. One day some of the popular girls turned on me and started spreading rumors about me. The next day I had literally no friends. I would walk through the halls holding my shorts so that the girls wouldn't "pants" me. I was thrown in the dumpster, my locker was regularly vandalized, and I would hide in the teacher's room during lunch hour. This went on for a year. Of course, I didn't reveal this to my parents because I was ashamed and simultaneously scared that they would try to help and the people who bullied me would get in trouble, which would make things worse for me. I learned to hide my fears, and I learned to protect the people who hurt me. *I wasn't good enough for girlfriends.*

This limiting belief was reinforced when I found a group of tough guys to protect me—a "gang," also called a "crew," where I lived in Los Angeles. They took care of me, picking me up from school and teaching me how to dress like a tough girl. I didn't do anything bad; I just hung out with them, like a pet. I started dating one of the main guys. He really wanted to have sex. He told me that he loved me. I told him I wasn't ready and wanted to wait until I was at least sixteen. A few weeks before my birthday he decided it was time. He wasn't violent with me, but he didn't listen to me. The next day he disappeared. He had another girlfriend. He didn't love me. I learned that my voice didn't matter and that "I love you" wasn't worth much. *I wasn't good enough for love.*

After college I was married to a really nice guy, but it wasn't right. We quickly divorced, and I fell for a man who needed me, and I equally craved him. When I found out that he was cheating on me and he told me that

I was horrible in bed, I made it my mission to be amazing in bed. I went to the bookstore and bought every book on sex and oral sex that I could devour. I put myself out to be the "perfect girl" and started following "the rules" of superficial dating. Shortly thereafter, I met a really great guy who asked me to marry him within three months, and I felt so lucky to be good enough to be loved again. But we didn't know each other, and soon it was very obvious that we were very different people and that our expectations were not aligned. To dodge dealing with it, I threw myself into my work. At the age of twenty-five I sold my second book and was writing for almost a dozen magazines. But my avoidance didn't fix the marriage, and so we ended it.

The thought that I was not good enough was reinforced by a boyfriend I started dating immediately after my divorce. Yes, *my second divorce.* An emotional mess and ashamed of the fact that I failed yet another marriage, I wasn't ready to be with this man, but he fascinated me and quickly I fell obsessively in love with him. He was a drug to me. I was addicted to him. But as addiction-based relationships go, it was fireworks followed by fighting. To say it was tumultuous would be an understatement. He told me that he was going to break me down so that he could build me up as a "better person." Then he rejected me in a way that I am uncomfortable writing about. But I am very aware of the damage it did. We broke up and I shut down completely. I wasn't good enough.

Just a few months later I met a guy who seemed to be my knight in shining armor (I write about him in a later chapter). He was extremely wealthy, and he made me feel like I was a princess as he lavished me with beautiful things . . . because he wanted to make me over into "someone better." I guess I still wasn't good enough despite the last guy's makeover. I was already emotionally weak and had little fight left in me, so I let him. He had lots of changes that he wanted to make. It started off with little biting comments—"Your laugh is so obnoxious." "You're such a bad kisser." "Are you sure you want to eat that?" "Those exercise pants make you look fat." "Don't you ever have anything interesting to talk about? Maybe you should start reading the newspaper every day so you can have a substantive conversation." Then he started pointing out my cellulite in the mirror, informed me that my job as a writer was just a cocktail conversation career and "encouraged" me to quit, told me that I made people feel uncomfortable when I was out at social events and that I should edit myself, pointed out that I had no style and literally threw away all but ten items of my clothing—which I bargained to keep. He told me to be presentable with my hair and makeup done at all times (except when working out), to read the newspaper before he came home and pull out five talking points for dinner conversation, and to lounge around in lingerie after dinner. The more I did what he said, the less we fought! When I was dressed—hair and makeup put together when he came home from work—he was happy with me. But I felt like a wild horse being broken into a circus act, ready to put on a show! And I horrifyingly sat back and watched as I lost myself, turning into that "yes girl" that I never thought I had the capacity to be, accommodating him in every way I could. I wanted to create a bubble around him so that he was always happy—like a bouncy house, nice and safe. It was my job (literally in some ways) to shield him from the real world, and I was responsible for making his life more enjoyable, sometimes to the detriment of my own enjoyment, as I was too concerned about his happiness to experience happiness myself. I learned to not voice my opinion and to put the needs of others first in order to avoid arguments or uncomfortable conversations. I know it seems like I'm painting an awful picture of him, and there truly were wonderful elements of our relationship, but it's often the stabs and jabs that stick. When the relationship finally ended several years later, I was a shell of a person, a house of cards. I was completely shut down. Since *I wasn't good enough,* I hid myself away in a cell deep within me, where no one could touch or hurt me again.

It was time to reinvent myself! After months of being too weak to leave my house, I further perpetuated the belief that I wasn't good enough by embodying Super Laurel. My heart was sealed, and no one could see through the façade that I put up. I wasn't going to let anyone hurt me again. Super Laurel had a big personality! She was witty, fun, spontaneous, sexy, and always interesting, with lots of stories to tell. But more than anything else, Super Laurel was beautiful and always "perfect." The first time I went out as Super Laurel, I was able to pull in the hottest, most eligible guy in the room. It was that night that I realized I had harnessed the power to get guys to want me. I became a player—like that hot guy who loves them and leaves them. It's not that I was trying to hurt these guys. They were really amazing people, and, when they showed interest in me, when they thought that "I" was good enough, I ate it up! I just wanted to be wanted, because more than anything else I wanted to be loved. The problem was that, just beneath the Super Laurel surface, I was numb. While these amazing men were sending love to me, my force field blocked those emotions so that I couldn't feel them. It also made it so that I couldn't love back. One guy after the next fell for me and wanted to see me a lot—all the time! Despite being in complete control, I was also a pleaser, and I would let them have as much of me as they wanted. But I didn't have very much to give and I quickly felt depleted and empty. And then, after a few weeks or maybe a couple of months of me giving all of me to them, I ended it. I had nothing left.

Years later that limiting belief was reinforced when I got back with the man who I had been obsessed with—the only man who had really ever tapped into my heart. He was my Achilles' heel. Again we were tumultuous—on and off and on and off. I kept leaving him because I wasn't getting what I needed from him: love and vulnerability. Each time I left, he walled himself up even more, became increasingly angry and resentful, and he trusted me with his heart even less. But we were both obsessed with each other. Despite getting back together, he told me that I didn't deserve his love, that I was a horrible and selfish human being, and that I had to prove myself worthy of his love for him to really open up to me again. We were spiraling in a seriously sick and toxic cycle, but for some reason neither of us wanted off the ride. Regardless of how "horrible a human being" I was, he wanted my body and my company, and he kept me around at an emotional distance, only occasionally letting his fortified guard down and being with me—laughing like we used to, which was what I so desperately craved. I felt like I was starving to death. He was right there in front of me, he was holding my hand, taking me out to dinner . . . but I couldn't access him. It was like dating a freezer or a brick wall. When I finally left—for good this time—I actually thought I was going to die. I felt that my heart had been ripped out of my chest. I immediately had a temperature of 103.5 and refused to leave my house, preferring to soak in the bath until the water was cold, then lay on the floor cuddling my dog for warmth.

After that, *I was done with this love bullshit.* I wasn't going to be hurt again—despite the fact that I desperately wanted love. I am a pathetic romantic and still believe in the fantasy of a fairytale love. But I had nothing left in me. So I pulled out my Super Laurel again. She is amazing! Men love her! She is always in control . . . As long as she stays perfect—perfectly put together, perfect in bed, and always very interesting and enticing. She is the ultimate seductress. Plus, she doesn't feel pain. She also doesn't feel love.

I was too afraid to let anyone see me, the real me, because my limiting belief of not good enough had so deeply rooted itself. But I was lonely and sad and missing love. In moments of extreme lows, I would want to go back to my Achilles' heel, because at least I knew that with him I was able to feel. My heart never closed to him, just to everyone else. I wanted to love someone else. I wanted to love someone else who loved me. The real me. Not the "me" who I put out when I was "on."

Why are those limiting beliefs serving you?

Those limiting beliefs are serving me because no one can hurt me again, because I don't let anyone see the real me.

Those limiting beliefs are serving me because I am in complete control of my feelings and therefore my life.

Why are you angry at those limiting beliefs?

I'm angry at those limiting beliefs because they are keeping my heart shut off and keeping me from truly experiencing love. Because I can't feel. I am numb. And I hate it.

Why are those limiting beliefs making you sad?

I'm sad because I feel alone. I'm sad because I feel like no one really knows me.

I'm scared that I am losing myself—my real self—because of my limiting beliefs. I am scared that if I continue to be a force field against love, I will never allow myself to be in a real and loving relationship again. I'm afraid that I will never again feel true and deep love.

Why do you regret your limiting beliefs?

I regret feeling not good enough because I believed it. And, because I believed it, I acted like I wasn't good enough. I stood for nothing, so I fell for everything. I was weak, but I pretended to be so strong. Believing that I wasn't good enough resulted in my shutting myself down. In shutting down I have shut out so many amazing people—both relationships and friendships. I regret creating a façade because in many ways even I started to believe that façade and I started to become Super Laurel. But people who truly know me—friends from my past—they can see through it, and they are disgusted by it. They want to see me. But I sometimes forget how to let her out of her cell. I regret that I didn't hold on to myself more fiercely. I regret that I didn't create a bottom line, that I didn't speak up for myself, and that I allowed myself to slip away. I believe that, had I actually been me—the real me—I wouldn't be alone. I think that, had I just been me and not the "me" that I put on, had I allowed myself to be the vulnerable and real me, I would have shown more integrity, and I wouldn't have contributed to the destruction of my relationship with my Achilles' heel. I regret believing in the make-believe that I created.

Why do you forgive yourself for your limiting beliefs?

I forgive myself for my belief that I am not good enough because I didn't have the tools to handle the pain of rejection and hurt on my own. I was too young to understand. When I was older, I was living in a fantasyland. I so badly wanted love that I would do anything to have it. And that desperation led me to act in a manic, insecure, and frantic manner that was not who I am. I forgive myself because I was acting out defensively. I forgive myself for believing that I wasn't good enough. I am good enough—the real me is good enough. It's the fake me that isn't, because that's superficial and fleeting, which is why I kept fleeing relationships.

How are you going to break free from your limiting beliefs?

I am going to break free from feeling not good enough by establishing bottom lines that create a safe environment for the real me to come out. Baby steps. With each step, as I feel more comfortable, I can adjust the boundaries.

I am going to break free from feeling not good enough by not always being what people want me to be and feeling like I always should accommodate others, including within my personal space. I know my tendency is to then feel crowded, which triggers me to be avoidant and to shut down.

I am going to break free from feeling not good enough by not running away when I allow someone to see a glimpse of me. I am going to allow people to love me for me, even if it feels uncomfortable and scary to be me.

I am going to break free from feeling not good enough by being true to myself, listening to my needs, and not being "on" in real life.

I am going to break free from feeling not good enough by being truly vulnerable, as opposed to the false bottom that I show people—making them think that they are seeing the real me.

I am going to break free from feeling not good enough by not being so hard on myself when I make little mistakes.

I am going to break free from feeling not good enough by being honest with others about how I feel, what I need, and how they can be there for me, instead of always shutting down their offers or not asking for help. My needs are not a burden.

Write a mantra that you will repeat every morning when you wake up that helps to reinforce this new healthy belief.

I am worthy of love. I am good enough to be loved. I will feel love for another. I deserve to be in a mutually loving relationship with a wonderful man who loves me for me. Here I am.

Dear Laurel,

You are good enough. You are worthy. You are deserving. You are a good person with a big heart and so much love to give. You love so hard it hurts sometimes. But you have been hurt too. And because you were hurt, you lost trust and sometimes you lost yourself. Sometimes you turned into a chameleon, trying to be what you thought you were supposed to be, do what you thought you were supposed to do, and behave how you thought you were supposed to behave. But that's not you. You were acting. And you don't have to act anymore. You are safe.

You will still be loved just by being you, even if you are being kind of a bitch sometimes. You don't have to carry all the weight. You don't have to be perfect. You don't have to be or do anything. Just be you. Do you. Here I am.

I am so sorry I let you down by not standing up for you. I am so sorry that I didn't voice your needs. I am so sorry that I ignored your intuition. I am so sorry that my knee-jerk responses ended up getting you hurt, as well as hurting others. We didn't have the tools. We didn't know. We didn't have the experience. We didn't have the confidence. But we do now.

I need you to know that you are not your worst actions. You are not your worst words. You are not your worst behaviors. You are not a bad girl, a selfish girl, or a bitch. You are a good woman who was weakened by circumstances that were out of your control, and as a defense mechanism you erected that Super Laurel wall as self-protection because you didn't know what else to do other than fight or hide. But you don't have to do that anymore.

Laurel, you are lovable. Laurel, you are loved. Laurel, you can and you do love others so deeply and so completely, and that's a good thing. You don't have to hide or defend anymore. All you have to do is be true to you, act how you feel, say what you mean, and know that you are worthy of friendships, of success, of happiness, and of love. I love you, Laurel. I love me. Here I am for the world to see.

xx

Love,

Me

Since then, I have been able to build up the back and of myself the substance behind the Super Laurel exterior. I have become strong in my core values, had the confidence to get raw and share my vulnerable and real self. And that's when I became truly overwhelmed by my power. Because I had even more! I'm not going to lie and say it was easy to switch back over, exposing myself again. It was a decision that I had to continue to remind myself of. Each time I felt myself floating away and the numb feeling taking hold, I had to focus on grounding myself, resisting the old comfortable habit of hiding and not feeling. With practice I was able to integrate the real me with the Super Laurel—toning her down just a bit and bringing her to life—real life.

* * *

NOW IT'S YOUR TURN

- Why are you single?
- What limiting belief is holding you back from meeting a great guy?
- Maybe you met a great guy—lots of great guys—but for some reason you can't seem to get past the fourth, or even the second, date. Or maybe you started dating a great guy, but then you put up derailing roadblocks, and you watched yourself as you sabotaged something that could have been really great.
- What story are you telling yourself?
- Are you afraid of failing or not getting what you *really* want, so you protect yourself by saying that you don't actually want it?
- Are you afraid of succeeding and finding true and deep love, but you don't believe that you deserve it?
- Are you too fat?
- Are you too skinny?
- Too ugly?

- Too damaged, messed up, and broken?

- Too busy?

- You're not worthy?

- Too scared for anyone to see the real you?

- Afraid you will have to change?

If any of the above ring true, or any others that I didn't list, you're not alone. I am going to take you down a staircase into the basement of your limiting beliefs. I want you to fully feel every emotion around it and go through a grieving process of letting it go. The reason it's a grieving process is that you have likely been living with this belief, this story, this occupant in your mind—which has taken over your life for a very long time. And now you're going to say good-bye.

But this staircase is in the shape of a U. It starts high, goes down deep to excavate the underlying emotions, then works its way back up to a positive place. I call this a U Strategy, and it's something that you will be using in various capacities—from removing blocks to flirting (which I will show you later—it's a fun one!). But, for right now, I need you to take a deep breath. I mean deep! This is a cleansing belly breath. Now let it all go like a gust of wind through your mouth. With a clear and open mind I want you to start writing the following things down. If it helps, listen to depressing music to get you into the place that opens your heart so that you really start to feel. This is my depressing playlist, and it's what I used to tap into my heart and make me feel when I was writing my personal U Dig, which you just read above:

- "Silent All These Years" (Tori Amos)

- "Say Something" (A Great Big World)

- "Same Mistake" (James Blunt)

- "Goodbye My Lover" (James Blunt)

- "Run" (Snow Patrol)

- "Possession" (Sarah McLachlan)

- "My Addiction" (Corn Ilana)
- "Jar of Hearts" (Christina Perri)
- "I Really Want You" (James Blunt)
- "Hide and Seek" (Imogen Heap)
- "Fall for You" (Secondhand Serenade)
- "Fake Plastic Trees" (Radiohead)
- "Delicate" (Damien Rice)
- "The Cave" (Mumford & Sons)
- "The Blower's Daughter" (Damien Rice)
- "Wrecking Ball" (Miley Cyrus)
- "Without Your Skin" (Keaton Simons)
- "Touch Me Fall" (Indigo Girls)
- "This Year's Love" (David Gray)
- "Someone Like You" (Adele)
- "Stubborn Love" (the Lumineers)
- "Sometime Around Midnight" (the Airborne Toxic Event)
- "Hallelujah" (Jeff Buckley)
- "Now Comes the Night" (Rob Thomas—this is a major tearjerker!)

Now open the door to your limiting belief basement and let's start walking down the steps.

Write down your limiting belief.

Write down what your life would look like if
you let go of this limiting belief.

Write down where this belief came from and the events in your life
that reinforced the belief, cementing it into your mind as "truth."

Write down three to five reasons why those
limiting beliefs are serving you.

1. Feeling unworthy keeps me from opening my heart, which makes it so that no one can hurt me.

2. I love feeling unworthy because it keeps me single, which allows me to stay in control of my life and allows me to do exactly what I want, when I want, and I don't have to change for anyone.

3. Feeling unworthy keeps me single and depressed, which makes it so that my family and friends pity me and feel like they need to take care of me—which I secretly love.

For a second I want for you to feel anger toward your limiting belief. Write down three to five reasons why you're angry at your limiting belief.

1. Feeling unworthy is keeping me from being happy and confident, and it pisses me off that I feel powerless to this feeling.

2. I hate that I feel unworthy because I see so many people around me who are happy and I am always miserable.

3. I can't stand feeling like I'm not good enough no matter how hard I try to be great.

Write down three to five reasons that your limiting belief makes you sad.

1. Feeling unworthy makes me feel alone and scared all the time.

2. I'm sad when I fall asleep knowing that no one is thinking about me. And I am even more depressed when I wake up feeling like there is no point in getting up.

3. It makes me sad to always be the one who people pity, as they look at me with those "poor girl" eyes whenever I show up to a party or family get-together alone . . . again.

Write down three to five reasons that your
limiting belief makes you scared.

1. I'm scared that if I continue to feel this way, I will never find someone to love me.

2. I'm afraid that if I keep feeling unworthy, I will die alone.

3. I'm fearful that I have become that miserable person no one wants to be around anymore as I am pushing people away.

Write down three to five reasons you regret your limiting belief.

1. If I didn't feel unworthy, I wouldn't have pushed away my ex, who really did love me and did everything to show me. But I didn't believe him, and I got cold, shut down, and pushed his love away. I wanted him to see just how unworthy of love I am.

2. I wish I didn't feel unworthy because I would have someone in my life right now who loves me and proves to me every day just how worthy I am. I would even be able to take him to my little sister's wedding in a few months.

3. I regret letting this feeling of unworthiness take over my mind, my body, and my life as I have begun to treat myself like I am unworthy, gaining weight to protect myself and make myself look even less worthy and walking around with a scowl on my face. I don't want to feel this way anymore. It makes me miserable and I want to be happy!

Write down three to five reasons you forgive
yourself for your limiting beliefs.

1. I forgive myself for feeling unworthy. I know that it came from when I was with my first boyfriend. He told me that he loved me, but he cheated on me and then told me that he never really loved me because I wasn't good enough for him. I was worthy then and I am worthy now. He wasn't worthy of me, but I was too young to process that. I forgive myself for holding on to those thoughtless words and for allowing them to shape my life.

2. I forgive myself for going into my protective shell and not letting anyone in. I was protecting my heart in the best way I knew how—by shutting it down, because I didn't have the tools to do it any other way. But I am ready now to remove the armor because I am worthy.

3. I forgive myself for the mistakes I made in my past. I was careless and I hurt other people's hearts, but I didn't mean to. I was young and stupid. I wasn't being malicious. I am ready to stop torturing myself. I am ready to be loved because I deserve it.

> Write down three to five ways that you are going
> to break free from your limiting beliefs.

1. I will create a new belief. But this time it will be true—not a false story that breaks me down. Every time I hear my limiting belief come into my mind, I am going to silence that voice and replace it immediately with something loving. I will repeat that loving thing over and over again until the nasty voice shuts up! I AM WORTHY OF LOVE—that is the truth.

2. I will allow myself to be vulnerable and experience emotion without fear. I know that I am opening myself up to being hurt by opening my heart, but I am stronger and more resilient now. I won't let setbacks, rejection, or mistakes close me off to the world again. It feels good to feel good, and I am ready to feel that way again. It has been too long.

3. I will not be so hard on myself or others. I will accept and give love. I know that I deserve love, and I will allow myself to be open to receiving it.

I know . . . That was a lot. But there is just one more step that I'd like you to do to help reinforce the next steps and help firm up in your mind the fact that you are worthy and deserving of happiness, love, and an amazing relationship. It's the top of the U. I want you to write yourself a love me letter using the information that you learned from the U Dig Strategy. Be gentle and loving with yourself. Tell yourself that you deserve love, that your limiting belief is not a fact. Apologize for mentally tormenting yourself for so long, for beating yourself up inside, and for treating yourself so poorly when you deserve to be treated like a princess.

Don't be afraid to really love yourself here. That's the point. You have to love you first. Set the standard of expectation for how others should treat you by allowing yourself to accept that love and showing yourself how it feels—how it feels to feel good, worthy, respected, beautiful, and loved. This letter will help you to understand what you are worth and open your heart so that you can receive love from others—and then you will be able to give love from a place of confidence. Sign it, "Love, Me."

SILENCING THAT BROKEN
RECORD IN YOUR HEAD

When you hear that voice in your head, the one that is silencing you, perpetuating the belief that is holding you back and strapping you down . . . What is it saying? Be honest:

- Do you believe it to be the truth? Or is it actually true? Because there's a difference. You may *think* it's the truth. But, really, is it true?

- Whose voice is it? Yours? Your mom's? Your ex's? A teacher's?

- How are your stories serving you?

- What are they protecting you from?

- What are you afraid will happen if you stop believing them?

- When will you be ready to let them go?

- How about now?

That broken record in your mind that keeps you down, that keeps you small, that keeps you stuck—that's your limiting belief. It's also called shame. I know, "shame" is a scary and dirty word that no one wants to think about, let alone say or admit to. We don't want to acknowledge it as something we are experiencing because it reveals true weakness and ultimate vulnerability. In fact, we often don't even know we are going through it, because it is something that is so rarely talked about. But here's the thing: if you don't speak it, it will eat you alive.

Let me clarify what shame is. It's the thinking that I'm not good enough, I'm an idiot, I'm not pretty enough, I'm stupid, I'm bad at my job, I'm not qualified, I'm an imposter, I'm a bad person, I'm a bitch, I'm a bad mom, I'm selfish, I'm too fucked up, I'm flawed, I'm a failure. . . . It's a labeling system. It's personal. It's taking ownership of a bad quality. Shame is brought on by fear—fear of losing love or connection—and it's perpetuated by silence and judgment. You fear that if anyone finds out that you're X, then you will lose connection, acceptance, and love. Or maybe you don't even think you deserve it.

When we feel shame, we act in ways that are not true to who we are. We lose control. Some of us want to get out from under that shame immediately, so we blame, or we rationalize it away. Some of us become avoidant. Some of us become overachievers; some of us self-sabotage. We react! We don't think. We do. Overall, we react in one of three knee-jerk ways: fight, flight, or freeze.

FIGHT

This means fighting back. You might turn it into blame—which could be why you're so judgmental of others or feel like you have an anger problem. You push back, you fight, you overcompensate with strength so that others can't see your "weakness."

FLIGHT

Flight is disappearing. You hide. You don't want anyone to see it, so you don't let anyone see you. You drop out, become flakey, a hermit; you sleep all the time or numb out. Numbing out can be mindlessly drinking too much, eating too much, shopping too much, or zoning out in front of the TV.

FREEZE

You feel like you are walking on eggshells, doing absolutely anything you can to make people like you, overcompensating for what's "wrong" with you by being extra, super, over-the-top good!

You might experience one reaction during certain times and another during others. The thing about shame is that it doesn't make us want to be better or change long-term. It just leads us to a knee-jerk reaction in the moment. It's not productive. It's destructive.

But here's the interesting thing: you aren't born feeling shame. It's learned. It might have started with your parents saying, "You're a bad girl." It may have come from a boyfriend, a teacher, or a "friend" saying, "You're stupid," or, "You don't deserve to be with a nice guy." Shame is also feeling like you're not allowed to be afraid, weak, imperfect, or not nice if you want to belong, be accepted, or be loved.

Shame is different from guilt. While shame is "I'm a bad person," guilt is "I'm a good person, but I did a bad thing that doesn't align with who I want to be." While shame is personal, guilt is situational. In other words, shame is "I'm a failure." Guilt is "I failed, but I'm not a failure." Guilt propels us to change behaviors and be more self-aware of our future words and actions better aligning with who we are as people.

So how do you overcome shame? You first have to acknowledge it. Call it out. Bring it out of hiding from its shameful place and to the surface. Then you need some empathy. While silence and judgment exacerbate shame, empathy—both from yourself and others—shrinks it. That's exactly why I had you do the U Dig Strategy.

Here's the thing though: when you bring attention to shame, when you expose it, it's hard to hide it again. Instead, it's time to start processing it by being aware of your triggers and your reactions in each situation, and preparing yourself to respond differently. Awareness and preparation are key, because if you fall for the trigger and fall into shame, you lose control and have a hard time thinking clearly enough to take it back. It won't be easy. But it will be worth it. True change only comes from bloodshed or tears. And with tears comes truth.

Personally, I had a realization of shame that felt like a smack in the face. I was shooting a reality television show as a dating and confidence coach in Kansas. I was working very long days, living in a Residence Inn for six weeks. I was away from everything that was familiar, I didn't have my dog, I was too tired and emotionally drained to talk on the phone with friends and family, and I didn't have much time to eat, so I pretty much lived on Balance Bars and energy drinks. While on-camera, my job was to be perfect—perfect looking (requiring pancaked makeup in Midwest summertime heat), saying perfect things, and being the perfect coach to this amazing girl whose life was changing before my eyes because of the intense emotional and physical work that we were doing together. Literally everything I said and did had an impact and was recorded by a microphone attached to the inside of my dress and at least one, if not two, cameras following me around. In addition to working sometimes sixteen hour days, during my few moments of downtime, I was also coaching clients over the phone and Skype and writing magazine articles and books. I had nothing left in me. When I wasn't on-camera, coaching clients, or writing, I was terrorizing myself by hypercritically analyzing my actions and behaviors, digging into my character, and breaking down every life mistake I had made in an attempt to extract strength from my weakness and transform it into a lesson. I wanted to be the best coach I could be, which required me to be my best self first. Simultaneously, I was communicating with my Achilles' heel, a man who was anything but complimentary of me and quick to break me down, highlight my failures, and shred my self-worth. Sometimes he would be yelling at me as I drove to the set, telling me what a disgusting and miserable human being I was. Tears welled up in my eyes and I hung up on him, then turned on for the camera—ready to inspire and empower this amazing girl who looked up to me completely. Thankfully, I was awesome at compartmentalizing. I put away the emotional abuse, knowing that I could pick it up later that night when I got home. And I was even better at erecting my "impenetrable" armor with an endless supply of strength and smiles.

To say I didn't sleep much would be an understatement: I was completely sleep deprived and emotionally weak. Despite the on-camera exterior, I was breaking down inside. And then I finally broke. I have always been that person who can handle everything—all at once! And I never asked for help. Friends and acquaintances thought I lived this fabulous life (thanks to Facebook). I had lots of friends, I was writing books, I was writing for magazines, I was appearing on TV shows, I was traveling to fancy places, I was eating at amazing restaurants. I did it all. I was everywhere. All the time! And I felt like I had to live up to the expectation of the life I portrayed for public consumption. I didn't want to let anyone down. So I continued to juggle all the balls . . . until I could no longer hide that they were dropping. Yeah, a lot was going on. Too much. I felt like a half-assed writer, a shitty friend (as I always flaked on plans and never showed up for anyone when they needed me), a bad mom to my dog, an awful girlfriend, as I was emotionally nonpresent and I was not taking care of my body. I was spread so thin that I had only the smallest doses of me to hand out, which, in the end, left nothing for me to refuel.

In the midst of shooting this show, I couldn't keep it together anymore, and I was washed over by shame, like a tidal wave suddenly appeared and hammered me down and held my head underwater. I couldn't hide from it anymore. Shame was drowning every area of my life, and I had to address it. There was no other choice. So I texted about a dozen friends, telling them how ashamed I was of my behavior and acknowledging what a shitty friend I had been. Some of them responded saying, "You're right, you have been a really shitty friend," which didn't feel good but was deserved. And then there were the ones who said something along the lines of "Are you okay? I appreciate you saying that. I also know that you're going through a lot right now. Focus on your work. Don't stress over this. Know that I love you and we will talk about it when you are back." One of my friends called me. She had been a friend since I was fourteen and knew me to my core. She wanted to talk about was going on in my mind. But the most powerful thing she said was "I haven't seen this side of you, this real, vulnerable, honest side of you since high school. I missed you. Now I remember why I have always loved you so much. Thank you for being vulnerable with me. Thank you for finally being human again." And that's when it hit me. I didn't have to wear my façade anymore. People liked ME more.

Once my shame was on the surface, I had to do something about it. I realized that I couldn't take on so much—which included work, friends, and even trips. I needed to make real, substantive changes in order to evolve into my best self. I had to be honest when it came to how much I could truly handle and juggle at once. I also had to admit to weakness and ask for help for the first time in a long time. I wasn't a burden as long as I was in equal (as opposed to what had been for me historically one-sided) relationships, where my friends were there for me, but I didn't show up during their moments of need. It was time for me to be equally there for them.

So let me ask you: What is shameful to you? What are you afraid of? What are you hiding? Why are you hiding it? Maybe you're afraid of being exposed, rejected, of people seeing that you're actually really fucked up beneath your "perfect" mask, that you can't do everything, you haven't achieved as much as you "could," you're a fraud, and you're not good enough.

But what is enough? As a society we are so hyperaware of "not enough," focusing too much on the negative rather than the positive. We don't get enough sleep, we aren't thin enough, we don't make enough money, we haven't achieved enough in life, we don't spend enough time with friends, we don't get enough vacation time. So when is enough, enough? We feel like we have to do it all, all the time. Like we have to be tough, resilient, and impenetrable. We hide our femininity for fear of it revealing weakness. But what is truly weakness? Showing our humanity or hiding?

According to research, femininity is conventionally defined as thin, nice, modest, pretty, and appropriate . . . And we wonder why we experience shame? We wonder why we feel too big or why we focus on the superficial? We wonder why we feel like we can't be ourselves?

Beyond how we view ourselves, who we choose to date has a lot to do with our shame triggers. We choose men based on that shame record that plays in our brains. We choose men who reinforce the stories in our minds.

I have done it too. When I was in elementary school, I had a math class that I was really struggling in. Despite the fact that I knew I failed this one test, when the teacher passed our graded tests back, I had an A. Later that day she took me into the hall and told me that I was too pretty to have to study and that I would meet a very rich man one day who would take care of me. I was completely offended and wanted to prove to her that I was smart and didn't need a man, or anyone for that matter, to take care of me! I could do it myself.

But not even realizing it, that conversation had implanted itself in my man-picking DNA, making wealth an essential element to any guy who had real potential. If a man wasn't rich enough for me, I either immediately dismissed him, or I constantly stressed in my mind that I wasn't living up to my potential.

It's time to retrain your brain. After all, what do you do with a broken record? You throw it away and get a new one. The old one was good for a while. It served a purpose. Maybe it protected you from opening up and therefore being hurt. Maybe it gave you the opportunity to have a lot of fun so that you would be ready to get serious . . . now. But it's not serving you anymore. In fact, it's hurting you. It's going against your ultimate purpose and not allowing you to experience the happiness that you truly *do* deserve. Let's replace that broken record. But let me warn you, it's not going to be easy. You have been listening to that same voice in your head for years, maybe even decades. Its message has ingrained itself in your brain and manifested throughout your life. Be gentle, understanding, supportive, patient, and compassionate with yourself as you make the shifts, tweak your thoughts, and eventually change your message and therefore your life. Change your mind, and your life will follow.

CHAPTER 2

What Do You Need?

Admit it: you want to be adored. You want to be put on a pedestal. You want your guy to love you and think you're amazing—just the way you are. You also want him to support you and encourage you to ascend even higher so that you can be your best, most radiant self. Instead of being intimidated or threatened by your success, he is proud of you, even shows off about his high-value woman. Your awesomeness inspires him to be the best he can be too. Your mere presence in his life infuses him with more confidence than he has experienced in a long time, as he works each day to prove his worth to you.

But you don't want to be looking down on your man. You want to be looking up at him too! You admire him. You learn from him. You are empowered by him. His presence in your life is a daily injection of inspiration to push your limits and achieve more and be happier than you ever thought possible.

What you want more than anything else is mutual adoration. You are both on pedestals. You are looking up at him. He is looking up at you. And together you are holding hands.

STOP LOOKING FOR WHAT YOU WANT AND GET WHAT YOU NEED

I knew what I "wanted." And I got him! He was handsome, quirky, funny, interesting, multifaceted, athletic, tall, smart, we had amazing chemistry, he made me feel like a princess, and we had great sex! He was also really, really rich. Like, money is no object rich. I'm talking Maserati, Ferrari, multiple houses (staffed with staff), and paintings by Picasso, Chagall, and Kenneth Noland hanging on the walls. And I'm not talking one or two. On almost every wall of his 14,000-square-foot house hung a piece of art worth more than most people's houses. The first time I entered the main home, I literally thought, "I could never live here. This place is like a museum." Six months later I was moving in. But it wasn't the money that I was attracted to. It was the man. He was so many things that I wanted!— yes, including the money. I mean, really, what girl doesn't dream of dating a multi-multi-millionaire? It's a fantasy, right? On our third date he took me on my first major shopping spree, and I swear I felt like Julia Roberts in *Pretty Woman.* Dior, Prada, Gucci—we hit them all, and he just started pulling clothes off the rack and sending me into the dressing room to try on the most beautiful dresses, skirts, sweaters, shoes, gowns, slacks, blouses, and bags. "She'll take that, that, that, that, that, that," he would say. "Send them to our hotel." He would drop his black card, and we were off to the next boutique. It was overwhelming—so much so that I went into the dressing room of Dior and started crying and called my mom to tell her what was going on. But they weren't tears of joy. Those tears were a mixture of dizzying emotions—excitement, insecurity, unworthiness, thrill, confusion, and joy! In this highfalutin atmosphere it would not be acceptable to emerge from the dressing room with mascara-darkened tears streaming down my face, so I quickly wiped my face, retouched my lashes, and pinched my cheeks, and when I walked out of the dressing room he pointed to a floor-to-ceiling photo of a bride dressed in a couture Dior gown and said, "That's what I will have designed for you some day."

I felt like Dorothy from *The Wizard of Oz*—swirling up in the air without any control. The fact that we shared a bottle of champagne at lunch on our way to the stores didn't help. It was like a dream. I mean, total package, right? He was everything that I wanted. And more! So why, after a few months of living in his museum of a home, was I unhappy? "Maybe I'm just homesick," I thought. After all, I had moved halfway across the country, and I was completely immersed in his unfamiliar world. So I started to try making some friends, taking dance classes, gardening, and establishing my own life—which he not only encouraged but pushed on me. Still, the façade of perfection started showing cracks, and we began to argue—a lot. We also drank—a lot, which definitely fueled the fighting.

He wasn't a fan of my career, which, according to him, was actually a job. "As defined in the dictionary," he would tell me, "a career is a regular paycheck or income stream, while writing is paycheck to paycheck— therefore, what you do is a job, not a career." Plus, according to him, it wasn't that interesting either. It was a "cocktail conversation" career with no real depth, no real importance, no real value to anyone. "If you want to be a real writer," he would say, "write a novel." After literally months of fighting about it, I had no more fight left and I quit. Feeling out of control, I used food as my comfort and started packing on comforting weight, which didn't go unnoticed—by either of us. The last thing I felt was sexy. In fact, I felt ashamed. Ashamed that I wasn't happier. Ashamed of my body. Ashamed that I didn't appreciate the life that he had given me. Ashamed that I quit my "job." Ashamed that I had somehow lost my voice, our regular screaming matches notwithstanding.

Okay, I am painting a really bad picture. It wasn't all bad. There were lots of great times too. He made me a priority and came home for lunch every day so we could eat and work out together, then came home early each night so we could drink wine as I finished cooking, then we would watch TV, talk about our days, take a bath, and connect. He encouraged me to be a more intellectual person and had me read the *Financial Times* each afternoon before he got home so that I would have "more interesting" things to talk with him about. And I actually did learn a lot despite my initial resistance and ongoing resentment. Anyway, I could go on and on, but the net net—a financial term he taught me and used in everyday life that essentially means "the value" or "the takeaway"—was that after almost three years it ended. I just couldn't take it anymore. I had become a shell of a person, and I missed me. So I gave up "everything," and, with only a couple thousand dollars to my name, I moved back to LA and was faced with reinventing myself, which included attempting to rebuild a career that I had ditched, remedy relationships that I had discarded, and rediscover myself again. What was so confusing was that I thought I had everything that I wanted. I did. But I didn't have what I needed—a man who loved, respected, and valued me (as opposed to the idea of me or the potential of what I could be).

* * *

Do you think, "I want a guy who is smart, funny, tall, handsome, sexy, interesting, well traveled, athletic, a foodie (even better if he can cook), has strong hands and loves giving massages, understands me, puts me on a pedestal, is good to my mom, loves my dog, has money (and is generous with it). . . . " And every time a relationship ends, you add to the wants to protect yourself from what your last guy lacked. It's endless, really. And although I appreciate that you have all of these desires that, combined, create a fantasy in your mind, I'm sticking a needle in that bubble because it's bullshit. It's fluff. It's fake. And—this might be surprising to you—it's unfulfilling.

You will never be satisfied if you continue to get only what you want. What do you actually need in a relationship? Once you shift from want to need, you will find that within your needs, you can also get what you want. But you have to change your focus first. Think about it this way—you might want to live on red velvet cupcakes. I mean, they are divine, right? But after a while you start to feel sick and you crave carrot cupcakes (or maybe a salad). What you realize is that, although you love red velvet cupcakes and when you first start eating one you feel like you could live off them, the fact is that you can't. They are amazing in small doses. But what do you actually need to survive?

Define your needs in a relationship. These are the things that your relationship needs to survive long-term. If it doesn't have these things, it is unsustainable and will die. Here are a few examples:

- Financial responsibility
- Kindness
- Family orientation
- Shared core values
- Communication
- Commitment
- Trust
- Emotional support
- Love
- Respect
- Showing up—emotionally and phsically

Now that is sexy! And more than that—it's relationship sustaining.

- Feeling sexy
- Seen and appreciated for being your true self
- Safe
- Interested and interested
- Mutual adoration
- Inspiration
- Intellectual stimulation
- Sexual compatibility

SCREW TALL, DARK, AND HANDSOME
(WHY LOOKS DON'T MATTER WHEN IT COMES TO TRUE LOVE)

My sister walked into her friend's bedroom and screamed. My boyfriend was naked on her wall—well, a poster of him. Yes, my first serious boyfriend was hot. I mean—smoking. So hot that he was a model for Abercrombie & Fitch—in their nude calendar. Yes, that hot. He hardly worked out, he ate homemade chocolate/coconut/pecan/marshmallow cream/caramel/graham cracker/peanut brittle seven-layer bars as regular snacks, and he still had eight-pack abs, those amazing "sex" muscles along his hip bones, the perfect V-shaped torso, and he played guitar. He had a chiseled face, green eyes, and was 6'2". He was a god.

And although he was unbelievably sweet and sensitive and we appeared to be the perfect couple, we lacked . . . Well, everything. We had nothing in common and nothing to talk about. We didn't share friends, activity preferences, lifestyles, or goals. But we certainly did have that sexual spark! In fact, the bed was pretty much the only place that we liked to be together.

I remember one day, about a year into our relationship, we were in the car driving onto the freeway when he looked at me and asked, "If you saw me driving next to you, would you think I was hot?" Without thinking, I replied, "No." He looked sad but didn't respond. Shortly thereafter we broke up because I realized that looks fade (no matter how hot they appear to be) and that lasting love is much more than skin deep.

* * *

Money, funny, blue-eyed blonde, tall, dark, handsome, cocky . . . What's your paper-perfect type? If you had to give points for importance to the following attributes, how would each rate: looks, intelligence, money, humor, sweetness, emotional availability, confidence, responsibility, respectfulness, understanding, supportiveness, communicativeness, fun?

Be honest—did you dedicate more points to looks than anything else?

Really, are looks more important than communication in the long term? After five years of being together, turn off the lights. Can you have a conversation? Looks deserve one point. Same as every other attribute. So stop being so intimidated by hotness. Stop allowing hair, eyes, height to dictate your next date. It's time to start paying attention to the things that actually matter in a man. If he's hot and rich too—that's a bonus! But it's not enough to base a relationship on.

If you create a perfect look in your head and then you just go after that look, you are blinding yourself to masses of men who truly could be your ideal match. *Especially* when that look that you love is hot!

YOU'RE NOT DATING A FACE; YOU'RE DATING A GUY

I know it's easier said than done, but you've got to look past looks. Looks fade. And really, so many things are so much sexier than looks. And I'm not even talking about a hot body! Ask yourself these questions:

- Can you sit alone in a dark room and talk with him for hours?
- Do you love who he is at his core?
- Could you spend two weeks stranded with him on an island? Cut out the sex stuff that is in your head. The reality is that after two weeks on an island without showers . . . not so sexy. Do you like to be with him as a person?
- Does he make you feel good about yourself?
- Does he inspire you to be a better person?
- Do you look up to him and respect him?
- Or are you just in awe of his Adonis body and cut-to-perfect face?

Because just skin deep is pretty shallow.

Now, that's not to say that you can't find real, deep, guttural, I-want-to-be-with-you-always love with a physically hot guy. If you find a hot guy who is also a fantastic human being, makes you feel like a priority, and is an excellent communicator—great! Just don't limit yourself to looks, or you could be settling for someone who really isn't right for you just because you want something pretty to look at. That, chickadees, is called arm candy. And you know what happens with just arm candy? You get bored, you crave something that's a little more meaningful and deep, and then you cheat (again—total generalization!).

ASIDE FROM LOOKS, WHAT ELSE CAN BE SEXY?

It's not that attraction is irrelevant. Attraction and sex appeal are very important! But what else, aside from a pretty face, can be considered sexy? A lot of things! Things that are ingrained in who he is. Things that grow rather than fade over time. How about ...

His core values: Who he actually is, at his core. What he stands for. We go in depth about core values in another section.

You admire him: You are proud of him. You look up to him. You learn from him. He inspires you to be your best self.

A secret smile: That side of the guy that is reserved only for you (or at least a select few). Sure, he may be outwardly somewhat geeky, seemingly closed off, a real jerk, or a shy guy, but the other side of him, the real side of him ... total opposite! Almost unrecognizable. Only you get to know the real him. You have this amazing secret.

His mind: Supersmart, witty, powerful, complicated men are fascinating! You could listen to them all day and night (and sometimes with that type of personality, you do).

He makes you laugh: Humor, someone who can laugh at himself, finds life funny, can instantly snap you out of a foul mood with his levity, makes you giggle, can leave you in absolute, tear-inducing hysterics. What a way to brighten your day—every day! Laughter isn't just the best medicine; it can be a major turn-on.

He's thoughtful: He comes over with cupcakes to celebrate even the littlest of life's ups and massages your neck on days you are down (without you even having to ask him to!). Even when he's out with the guys, he sends you the occasional text to tell you that he's thinking about you.

Confidence . . . almost to the point of cocky: He walks into a room and it lights up; people look, some even stare; he does not go unnoticed. But it's not because he's hot, loud, or obnoxious; it's because he has a confidence that is so strong it's hard not to notice. You feel taken care of when you're with him, safe, in good hands. He is proud, and you are proud to be with him.

You matter: Your opinion, your stories, your history, your preferences, your comfort, your health. You matter. When you're talking, he doesn't just listen; he engages, he asks you questions, he makes observations, he wants to know more. You are a priority, and he makes sure that you know it.

A feeling of home: Home isn't necessarily a location. It's a feeling. As much as I think "Home is where the heart is" is kind of a lame saying, it's true. The feeling of home is comfort, safety, the ability to walk around naked (physically and figuratively) and not feel insecure, total and complete trust, a foundation, a knowledge that he is coming back to you and you are coming back to him like a boomerang. It's being able to completely exhale. It's knowing that everything is going to be okay. Now *that* is sexy.

Each of us is attracted to different things. Some might find my turn-ons silly or even stupid. That's fine. What is attractive to you? Think about it. What intrigues you? How do you want to feel?

LOVE MAY BE BLIND,
BUT CHEMISTRY IS BLINDING

Your pulse starts to race, your face is flushed, your nerves stand on end, and you feel what you swear is a magnetic pull to his lips from the moment you shake his hand, make eye contact, or even just from the second you see him. When you kiss him it feels like you're taking a drug. You're dizzy, almost high. Your chemistry is off the charts. But that might not be a good thing.

Chemistry is that feeling of—being in love. I know, as intoxicating and tempting as it may be, the problem with chemistry is that you can be gravitationally pulled to the wrong person. In fact, chemistry triggers the exact same brain reaction as cocaine. It also triggers a similar physical reaction: the feeling of angst, sweaty palms, nervousness, a racing heart, crazy obsessive thoughts . . . Wait, how is this a good thing again? Here's the other interesting fact: it has been shown that chemistry wears off within eighteen to thirty-six months. And we wonder why the divorce rate is so high. Most couples are married within the eighteen- to thirty-six-month threshold—essentially under the influence of chemistry—and they don't take the time to get to know each other on levels deeper than the intoxicating rush before making the "till death" vow. Then the drugs wear off, and these two people suddenly wake up, look at each other, and realize, "I don't know you, and what I do know, I don't like."

There is a difference between chemistry and intimacy. Intimacy is love, and it develops and grows over time. It also endures. It is formed on a deeply rooted foundation of trust, understanding, honesty, and authenticity. Intimacy is the commitment to the commitment. That's not to say that you can't have both.

The danger of falling for just chemistry is that you are blinding yourself to the red flags, ignoring the danger signs, and choosing to overlook the fact that this guy is not good for you. He may even be bad for you. He is a trap, a test, a ploy to see whether you fall for the wrong guy again or whether you are ready to take responsibility; be on-purpose (meaning moving toward your goal) when it comes to your hopes, dreams, and future; and build a relationship with a man who is not only good for you and treats you well but a man who fulfills your needs and wants. If you're sick of being treated like shit, then stop succumbing to the superficial pull of the bad boys who don't adore you, don't make you a priority, and don't want a future with you; and start focusing on opening your heart to true and deep love with good guys who will not just treat you right but treat you amazingly well. Now, I'm not saying that you should shut down your sexual needs with Mr. Magnetic and settle for "Mr. Right" just because he's a good guy and he's crazy for you. What I'm saying is that you shouldn't fall for the quick fix, the instant high, the bad guy who will slay your heart and trap you in a drug-like state of fantasy.

So what are you supposed to do? Prequalify. By prequalifying your dates first, you have the opportunity to really get to know a guy before you go out with him, thereby affording yourself the opportunity to see whether he has the potential of being a true match—one who is good for you, good to you, *and* who is attractive to you. (It just might be a more gradual and less intense—at first build.) Or if he is made of red flags but just—and I really do mean just, as in *only*—so damn sexy. That guy—the so damned sexy guy who is bad for you and who you know from the get-go is never going to be able to be the guy you need despite the fact that you want him right now—is who you really should immediately knock off your list of potentials and not go out with. Because if you do, you risk getting wrapped up in the ecstatic rapture of *just* chemistry, and you are pretty much postponing your purpose: to find true and deep and real love and intimacy.

HOW TO BE ATTRACTED
TO THE RIGHT GUY FOR YOU

Take it from someone who was always looking for the "perfect" guy who is more, better . . . everything. Screw more and better; this is about who is best—for you. I've experienced a lot of really great guys in so many different ways yet always found a flaw that was detrimental enough that it warranted leaving. Take it from someone who has years (sometimes mere months) later regretted some of those brush-offs and breakups upon realizing that he really wasn't so bad after all and I made a decision to dump him too fast. In fact, he was pretty damned close to perfect for me.

As my dad said to me after one breakup with one of those pretty-damned-close-to-perfect guys, "Laurel, what does a guy have to do and be for you to realize how great he is for you? When will enough be enough? Or do you just believe that the grass is always greener?" I know, the grass could be greener, there might be someone better, and really the only way to find out is to go look. You don't want to sell yourself short. However, you also can't expect one guy to provide everything you need. And here's the thing: pass up on one guy because you aren't into his idiosyncrasies, and be ready to take on another's unknown shit that might actually be unacceptable to a successful relationship.

Realistically, think about this:

Women are ingrained at a young age with an attitude of abundance—essentially an attitude of confidence and the knowledge that there truly are plenty of fish in the sea and you can pull in as many as you'd like! In our twenties we aren't rejected as often, so we become picky—because we can. As we age, we carry that attitude with us and suddenly our expectations become unrealistic as we are constantly thinking that there is better, bigger, more, out there. Men are the opposite. When they are young they are often rejected, as age-appropriate women are going for older guys, leaving men with an attitude of scarcity. As men age, they don't have these crazy unrealistic expectations like we do. They don't think, "I like her, but that one little quirk annoys me so it's over." Reality check: guys of marrying age can date women of any age. Sure, you can too, but let's face it—your dating pool dramatically shrinks as you age, while a man's typically expands.

Now think about this:

1. Who have you dumped (or passed up on completely) for stupid reasons? But once he was taken, then engaged and married to a great girl, you questioned why you dumped him for such a dumb reason? I've done it. I ended it with a great guy who really had pretty much everything I needed AND wanted in a partner, because I felt like he was too close with his brother—who I didn't particularly like. Another guy was way too nice to me. He snores was my excuse with a really great catch. He just has no edge. The number of men I have said that about is way too long. His kissing style made me feel like I was getting intimate with a lizard. His car was so feminine that it made me look at him differently, fixating on all of his effeminate traits. And then they got married. All of them. And I was still single and wishing I hadn't fucked that one up. What about you?

2. What traits actually make a good husband? How about honesty, kindness, loyalty, commitment, communication, financial stability, emotional availability? Think back to your needs.

3. Are you fixating on guys who are unavailable? What about guys who would be great if . . . if you could fix them?

4. If you expanded your options, became an equal-opportunity dater, and took off your blinders, you would have *so many more* choices! Suddenly dating will be a blast again!

5. Stop looking for the negatives and instead focus on the positives. I know it's hard. You are essentially flip-flopping your perspective. Instead of thinking, "He's great, but . . . ," try to focus on what is actually great about him! *Now*, think about all of the guys you've fallen for—hard—who have been horrible for you. Did you fixate on the positives to make them fit your idea of perfection as you justified why you are interested in them just

because they're hot or rich? For all of those bad guys you finally realized (or not) were not a fit, create a list of negatives about them and fixate on those instead of the fantasy that they never did and never will live up to.

Remember: You can't see all the good men around you if your nose is stuck up in the air.

Imagine a cake. You've got frosting and cake. Both are essential for it to feel complete. You are that cake. Your dating purpose and your core values make up the bready cake. Your femininity, flirting, and X Appeal (which we will talk about later) are the frosting. Let's first bake the cake, then we can layer on the frosting.

When it comes to dating, what's your purpose? People date for three main purposes:

1. Having fun

2. Self-exploration

3. Finding the one

Are you dating for the purpose of having fun?

Maybe you are in the self-exploration and growth phase, and your purpose is expanding yourself, experiencing different people, places, and things so you can enjoy a more layered and dynamic life as you become more interesting and therefore irresistible.

Or are you ready to finally meet the one (as opposed to just another *some*one)?

Whatever your purpose is, be aware of it, and make choices based on the direction that you have decided to go. For example, maybe you're interested in just having fun, messing around, and enjoying a free-spirited attitude without any ties to hold you down. So why do you continue to be drawn to serious types who reel you in and plant you in a relationship that shortly thereafter makes you feel like you're suffocating and forces you to jump ship and break the poor guy's heart—over and over again?

Or is your purpose to enrich your life by dating fascinating men with diverse interests who encourage you to learn, explore, and experience hobbies, activities, and lifestyles that you hadn't been exposed to before. Yet you are repeatedly attracted to the same-guy-different-face whose habits and lifestyle are comforting because they don't challenge you. Or is your purpose to get into a serious relationship with a man who is in a secure and happy place in his life and is ready for a commitment; still you continue to date guys who are superficially fulfilling but are far from ready to really commit? Stop for a second and ask yourself, "Do my words and actions reflect my desired outcome?"

DEFINE YOUR CORE VALUES

I was once asked by a boyfriend, "Who are you?"

I responded, "I'm a writer."

He asked again, "No, who are you?"

"Um . . . ," I said, "I'm a writer."

"That's it?" he questioned.

Offended and defensive, I responded, "Is being a writer not good enough? Well then, who are you?"

"I'm a man of my word, I am a thinker, I am a perfectionist, I am a seeker of knowledge and truth, I am a business man, and I am a chef," he responded.

And then I got it. I am not my career. I am not my relationships. I am not my beliefs. I am defined by a combination of several core things. Core values. So I sat with myself and started to write down what those values are. I started with a list of twenty-five. Realizing that many of them fit within others, I consolidated the items in the list down to ten, many with subcategories. Then I began defining them in two ways: what each meant to me and what experience in my life made that value an essential—assigning an emotion-emitting experience to it. As I did this, I cut out three more values and assigned them instead as subvalues, bringing my core list down to seven. Seven pillars that defined me. Seven things that were essential to me, in me. Some of which were more aspirational at the time than actual, as I knew they needed more development. Seven values that when combined created my best self. Seven elements that if ignored or weakened within myself, I feel like something is missing or that I am being untrue to me. Seven musts in terms of what my future partner must share or at least honor in me. Immediately, something shifted inside me. It was a knowing, an understanding, a confidence in who I am and what I stand for, a daily focused purpose to improve and stand for each value as best as I could, as well as a more defined understanding when it came to what it was that I was looking for in a partner.

And what was interesting about defining my core values was that my boyfriend at the time, the person who put me on the path of defining these values of mine, didn't share who I was at my core, my #1 family. He wasn't close with his, and he wasn't sure he wanted one of his own. I also came to find out that he wasn't the understanding or forgiving type—my #2 core value. With a more fine-tuned awareness of myself and an evolved understanding of my needs, I began to realize that I was attempting to put my values on him, assuming that, because they were central for me, they must be essentials for him too. And that's when it clicked. They weren't. Our relationship had always been a lot of work. It was hard. It was littered with misunderstandings and communication gaps. I never felt that he got me or heard me—and he felt the same way about me. After trying to force a square peg into a round hole, it was painfully obvious that though we loved each other very much, sometimes love simply is not enough if you are two too different people.

LAUREL'S SEVEN CORE VALUES

1. Family

2. Understanding and forgiving

3. Deep love

4. Communication

5. Passion and drive

6. Balance

7. Learning and experiencing

* * *

Do you want to be a "total package"? Because you're not just pretty, just successful, just a mom, just a writer, *just anything*! You are who you are at your core, and *that* is what you lead with. If you lead with anything else, you are leading with something superficial, you are leading with your walls. It's the substance behind the wall—your castle—that is truly enticing and sexy. And that's what we are about to explore.

Before you are truly ready to find the right guy for you, you first have to take a real, deep, hard, honest look at yourself.

- Who you are?
- What's most important to you?
- Where do you stand when it comes to priorities in life?
- What do you stand for?

Your core values, the values that you will not budge on—they are your foundation. Once you are clear on that, you will better be able to decipher whether your potential guy's beliefs align with yours, whether you stand on the same ground.

Not sure who you are? Unclear as to what defines you? Do you sometimes feel like you are shapelessly floating? Or maybe you are numbly plowing through life on autopilot? Do you feel lost? When you aren't grounded within your core, you may feel like you're a tree running around carrying its roots, a butterfly helplessly caught in a windstorm, or a piece of clay taking on the shape that any warm thumb forms you into for now. Or maybe you just feel like you're missing something. Do you want to know why you feel this way? Do you want to know what you're missing? You're missing you. You aren't being true to your core values. You aren't being true to you. You have edited yourself out of the equation in order to be what you think you should or are supposed to be.

Not anymore. It's time to give you shape and define who you are. Because as Katy Perry says in her song "Roar," "I stood for nothing, so I fell for everything." Once you know who you are, what you stand for, and what defines you, you will have more confidence and a deeper understanding of your value. Self-worth starts with knowing yourself.

As I said, you are a castle. Your core values are the foundation on which everything else is built. They are your firm beliefs. Some of them may have been instilled in you by your upbringing, others from life experiences. They are deeply rooted and unwavering. To help you think about what your core values are, here are a few ideas (in addition to mine above). Notice that I have broken them down into four categories, reflecting the multiple sides of you. Try to choose at least one core value per category.

- Heart—compassion, love, respect, romance, understanding, affection, forgiveness, sensual, relationships, authenticity
- Head—law abiding, drive, integrity, commitment, truth, knowledge, confidence, loyalty, abundance
- Spirit—peace, happy, calm, balance, trusting, religion, optimism, spirituality
- Experience—enjoyment, fun, adventure, spontaneity, healthy, curiosity, home, personal growth, physical activity

Sit and think about what you stand for. If it helps, think about your family, your upbringing, the values that you were raised with. Do you still believe them? Have they altered for some reason? Have you created your own values based on experiences or personal awakenings and awareness that may have shifted your beliefs? Think about the elements that are important to you but are missing from your life. Just because it's a core value doesn't necessarily mean it's something that you actively practice, which might be exactly why you feel lost, inauthentic, empty, or like you are floating. When you are not following through or practicing, when you are ignoring or not being true to your core values, you may question your definition of self and worth. This isn't the time to judge yourself. It's time to tap in to your truth. If you are weak with one of your core values, that's okay. It gives you something to work on. You are on-purpose to strengthen the weakness within that value.

Remember, though, these are not values that you want your partner to have. This is all about you. This is your blueprint, your definition of self.

You might find that you start with a long list, then realize that many of the values are actually more like subcategories within another overarching value. Narrow your list down to seven.

Once you come up with your core values, plus the list of subcategories, write a paragraph description that helps define each value. For example, what does family mean?

Next, make it personal to you, and write why that value is central to who you are. What experience, feeling, memory, or belief contributed to its importance? How does each value appear in your life, and how do you embody it?

PURPOSE + CORE VALUES = YOUR BEST SELF

More than being on-purpose in love, you need to be on-purpose for each of your core values. Why? To embody your best self and therefore attract a great guy who complements, inspires, and empowers you, you need to be true to each of your core values. Examine your core values and subcategories list and think about the areas within each that are your weakness and that you need to strengthen. Here's an example:

Core Value: Integrity/Truthfulness

Subcategory: Trust, honesty, commitment

Weakness: I am not honest to myself or to others about my needs

Purpose: I need to check in with myself and make sure that I am being honest about how I am feeling, what my needs are, and whether they are being met. If they are not being met, I need to not be afraid to voice them, because *my needs are valid*.

Core Value: Compassion

Subcategory: Kindness, caring, nurturing

Weakness: Vulnerability. Compassion requires vulnerability, which I am afraid of showing for fear that if I let my guard down, I will be viewed as weak. I also struggle being compassionate with myself and have a hard time showing myself love and caring. I tend to be very hard on myself.

Purpose: To fulfill my core value of compassion, I need to know that true vulnerability takes a lot of strength and courage. It does not express weakness. Courage, at its root, is "core." I need to have the courage to speak my truth, from my core—my core values. I need to be kinder and gentler with myself, showing myself love and understanding instead of being so hard on myself. My self-judgment is a reflection of how judgmental I am of others.

Subcategory: Development, learning, changing, flexibility, openness, fun

Weakness: I am great at growth when it comes to my business. I am also taking courses to emotionally develop and tap into my heart. My weakness is having fun. Sometimes I don't even know what is fun for me. I am always so purpose driven that I forget to just let go and have fun! Part of the problem is that it takes vulnerability to truly have fun, because that requires me to let my guard down, laugh, and just be, and that scares me. I also feel like I don't deserve to have fun, or that I am wasting time because I am not yet as financially successful as I know I should and can be.

Purpose: I need to do things that allow me to get out of my comfortable but restrictive box. I will start signing up for classes like aerial yoga, ceramics, and even pole dancing in order to discover what is fun for me. I will also sometimes just go to the beach with my dog and run around on the sand. No agenda except to have fun. To be my best self, I know that I need to sometimes refuel myself through fun activities. I also know that having fun allows me to have a more positive outlook, and with a positive outlook I am more effective and efficient at my job.

Core Value: Authentic Love

Subcategory: Self-love, patience, forgiveness, understanding

Weakness: I neglect myself because I don't take the time to listen to my needs. I often feel like I am running a marathon and I am always behind. I'm not patient with myself. I am internally conflicted, as I am very understanding and patient at work but I don't practice it with myself. I often bite off more than I can chew, which results in feeling like a failure when I can't accomplish my goals. I too often overpromise and underdeliver, then I am ashamed of myself for not living up to my personal expectations.

Purpose: I need to slow down. I realize that I don't show myself love. I don't treat myself as I would treat others. If I allow myself to take on only as much as I can realistically deliver, I won't constantly feel like a failure. I need to take personal time to tap into, then take care of, my needs. I know that I am a better boss when I am fully fueled, as opposed to constantly running on empty. I also know that I am less likely to attract someone into my life if I don't carve out space to let someone in. I need to make myself the example of my expectations and model how I want to be treated in a relationship. I am a priority, and I need to first make myself the priority if I want to be treated like someone else's priority.

Core Value: Relationships

Subcategory: Priorities—1) Self, 2) Faith, 3) Future partner, 4) Family, 5) Friends

Weakness: I often put the needs and opinions of my family and friends over my own. Because my life is so full of social obligations, I don't have time for a future partner, and I know that's a turnoff to men. I feel like I have to fill every moment with plans and activities. The problem is that I'm always overwhelmed, tired, and left feeling empty at the end of the day. I never have time for me. I don't allow myself to refuel, which makes me feel like a half person with nothing left to give.

Purpose: Check in with myself, listen to what I truly need and want, and do that. Make time to just be. Stop doing, start being. Create time and space for my future partner. Think: Do my beliefs match my words, match my actions, match my purpose? Remember my relationship priorities.

Being on-purpose to strengthen your core values helps promote your relationship purpose because you can only be your best self, and therefore attract a great guy who is his best self too, if you are your true self. Your true self is formed within a strong foundation of core values. You are rooted in what you believe in and who you truly are. When you are on-purpose with your core values, your life has purpose.

ME TO WE

Now that you have started to figure yourself out, when you meet someone you think might have potential, think about whether your core values align. If they differ, can you still create a foundation together as one, with your two value systems complementing each other's to make you stronger? Or do the differences create a foundation too unstable to hold up under life's little earthquakes?

Think about it this way: you can be physically, chemically, and sexually addicted to someone, but if you don't like him, if he stands for things that you don't believe in, if he doesn't respect your values, if you are two totally different people at your core, well, sex, chemistry, and even love simply aren't enough. Define your core values. They are the root of your confidence and everything else that we are going to be discussing in this book.

INTENTION BOARD:
HOW DO YOU WANT TO FEEL?

I knew who I was, but my future was still fuzzy. I had no focus and no idea what I wanted to accomplish. Without direction, how could I take steps to move forward? So, with my core value pillars firmly in place, it was time to dive into feelings.

I had been emotionally burned. And it was partially my fault. I had lost my way, forgot my focus, ignored my needs, and become a bit of a chameleon in an attempt to be the person I thought my boyfriend at the time wanted me to be. Honestly, I lost myself. I remember feeling myself slowly slipping away. At first I resented him for not acknowledging or listening to my needs. But then I dropped the resentment and pushed on as a partner in his life, infusing myself into his world. My friend Christina told me that she didn't recognize me anymore and distanced herself from me. I didn't understand. And then I did—and that's when I left him.

During the weeks after the breakup, I felt like I had been frozen in a block of ice. I didn't know how to act, what to say, who to be. Afraid of being inappropriate, awkward, or saying the wrong thing, I didn't leave my house. But the one thing that I did do was something that I had done years before as a fun and emotionally connecting and grounding pastime—making collages out of magazine clippings and photographs. I took the collection of magazines that I had stacked in a corner and clipped words and images that resonated with how I was feeling, but more than that—how I wanted to feel. I created a collage of emotions and intentions, and within those words and images I found strength. Every morning I would sit with my intention board and focus on a word, an image, an energy that leapt off the page, and I would remember that moment throughout the day. It became my daily driving force. And soon I found myself again, and then I saw my path in front of me, and I was able to begin to move forward.

The intention board isn't about creating a collage of images that you want your life to look like. It's about creating a collage of emotions and feelings that you want to extract the energy from and evoke in your life. On a poster board, place images and words cut from magazines, drawn, or written to illustrate the energy, feelings, and loose intentions of how you want your relationship to feel like. Think about your relationship needs, which we discussed at the beginning of this chapter. What does a relationship within which those needs are met feel like? How do you feel when you are on-purpose with your core values? Think about what love feels like to you, what family feels like to you, what turns you on, what makes you feel loved, what makes you feel comforted, what passion feels like to you, what home feels like to you, and what makes you feel safe. Unlike your core values, which define who you are, your intention board is how you want to feel.

Every morning as you are drinking your tea or coffee or eating breakfast, sit in silence with your board and just take it in. Look at the images, read the words, and imagine how the energy of that board, those desires, that feeling, can translate into your life. Don't take each image literally, just take its energy. Before you go on a date, spend five minutes looking at the board, focusing on the elements that pop out at you and remind you what truly is important to you—and important in the person you are looking for and the life you are looking to live.

With the intention of your board in mind, see how you can make small changes throughout your day to make those goals take shape.

Don't be attached to the form or outcome of your intention. You have to surrender a little bit of control here and trust that your intention will come true in some shape or form—just maybe not in the exact image you saw on paper or in your head.

GET A LIFE BEFORE YOU GET A BOYFRIEND

I fell for the Jerry Maguire line too:"You complete me." It's so romantic. But it's horseshit. It's more about "you balance me." You don't want him to be the center of your universe. In fact, that can destroy your relationship. The last thing you want to be is half of a whole, because that translates to being an incomplete person. And when it comes to relationships, two halves do not make a whole. They add up to an unhealthy, codependent, needy, and insecure duo. And that's not sexy, nor does it have longevity.

Feeling not so whole? Get a life. Here's how:

Be busy. Don't pretend to be busy. *Be* busy. Be independent, go out with friends, pursue hobbies and interests—have a life! One of the sexiest things a woman can be is interesting. You have experiences, opinions, and a perspective that you bring to the conversation and the relationship.

Be passionate. If you are passionate about your career, your projects, your classes, your *anything/something*—perfect! It shows him that you have this super passionate side, and that will make him think, "If she can be that passionate about *that*, I can't wait until she puts some of that passion on me!"

Be self-sufficient and autonomous. You can take care of yourself—financially and emotionally.

Become more interesting by expanding your interests, exploring yourself, and learning about other people and things. When you are interesting, you can contribute to high-quality conversations.

Have an opinion. But don't just have an opinion for the sake of hearing your voice. Voice your needs, wants, interests, insights, and preferences. Contribute to the conversation.

Share your experiences. Bring up the insight that you obtain while apart as fodder for your conversation. Share your experiences. Each time that you get out of your box and do something different, you are becoming a more layered, dynamic, and therefore attractive person. Let him in on your perspective. Expand his mind and enrich his life through yours.

This isn't to say that you should be an overly busy bee or a social butterfly. You don't want to make it seem like, although you might not be desperate for him, you *are* desperate to always be out and about. This isn't a competition to see how many friends or obligations you can juggle. This is about being a whole and content person on your own, with a life that is fulfilling. If that means spending high-quality time alone—great! Every hour of your day doesn't need to be filled up. In fact, even every day doesn't have to be occupied by something to do or someone to see.

More than what you bring to the table, being confident and fulfilled on your own dramatically decreases the chances that you will be needy—an instant turnoff for a guy. You don't *need* him. You want him. You have lots of exciting things to fill up your day, but you choose to make the time for him because he is a priority—not *the* priority, but *a* priority.

The idea is that without him you are complete. But life is richer together. And that's attractive. In fact, many men say that it's the most attractive trait in a woman. Sure you can be beautiful, fun, sweet, and successful. But what do you add to his life? What do you bring to the table that makes his day to day better because you're in it? If you're afraid that your layers may intimidate or scare him away, then you're going for the wrong guy. The fact that you're so incredible should make him proud; it may even make him want to ascend to your level as you encourage each other to be your best selves just because you are in each other's lives.

Get a life. Then find a great guy who appreciates your life. Soon your life will be even greater because of it.

GET REAL! FIRST DATE CONVERSATIONS:
FRAMING YOUR STORIES

Stop judging me based on what you see sitting in front of you. I am not that girl you've made me up to be in your head. I may have blue eyes, blonde hair, a magazine smile, and my body is wrapped in a nice curve-defining dress, plus the extra added flare of five-inch stilettos that make me appear 5'7" instead of 5'2". But what you see is not me. Sadly, many women allow their looks to define them. We also tend to judge others based on what's revealed on the outside. But strip me of my clothes, and what you'll see is my story, the winding path of experiences, emotions, and introspections that collectively create me. So what's my story? Well that's an entire book in itself. But I can frame out a few episodes that will give you a little taste of my spirit, of what thrills me, makes me feel happy and fulfilled, disappoints me, and what is my overall outlook on life.

I was in Finland a few years ago with a boyfriend. It was my birthday, October 4, and the temperature was freezing. And although I came carrying a suitcase filled with beautiful dresses, designer coats, and painfully stunning stilettos, we decided to head out to his summer house in a small town where the dress code is jeans, oversized puffy jackets, and black rubber boots. When we arrived at the house by a lake almost frozen, he set aside my suitcase and provided me with a pair of his mom's rubber boots and an old feather-filled jacket with a few holes burned by fire pit embers from sitting too close. He had an idea that he thought would be a fun way to spend my birthday. It was a surprise. A few hours later we piled into a small boat stocked with a cooler and two sleeping bags and headed off to a small, uninhabited island, maybe a quarter mile across, verdant with trees, moss, and berries. He instructed me to walk along the perimeter, collecting anything man-made that I could find, while he canvassed the area for the perfect campsite where we would stay the night.

Let me just pause here to tell you about the birthday trip that another ex had taken me on three years before. He surprised me and charted a 150-foot yacht, flew in ten of my friends to the Bahamas, and spent about half a million dollars on the most extravagant experience I could imagine, replete with an onboard chef, massage therapist, scuba instructor, evening fireworks shows—just for me. Bands were flown in for dance parties on various islands that he rented along our path, and an endless supply of caviar, truffles, crab legs, and rose champagne was available.

Now back to the campsite. During my perimeter walk, I discovered a glass bottle, a one-liter plastic bottle, and the remnants of what looked like a large cage to trap fish. He had found a campsite near the edge of an eight-foot drop-off to the lake, protected from the wind by a large boulder, with a flat-ish area adequate for us to both lie down. While he took the fish cage and started to construct a shelter, I set off again to collect wood from fallen trees so that he could build the fire. With a decent stockpile that I thought would sustain us through the night, I started gathering moss from the rocks, delicately lifting it in 8" × 10" sheets, trying not to rip nature's craftsmanship of two-inch-thick interwoven layers of pillows of green moss atop roots that held on to a thin layer of dirt. As if I was creating a patchwork blanket, I carefully laid each sheet of moss on the fish cage, constructing a solid cover.

Several hours later, as the sun was beginning to set, we had our fire and our shelter but no food. As if we had done this hundreds of times before, he and I just fell into a rhythm, a knowing of what was needed next. I set off to collect berries while he headed to the edge to fish. Handful after handful, I piled berries into a dimple in the boulder beside our campsite, until I was satisfied with my haul. Next I took the plastic and glass bottles and cleaned them as well as I could with my fingers in the lake, filled both to the brim, and returned to find him fileting a gigantic pike. The sun was showing its last flash of colors—red and orange across the sky—and before darkness overtook our home, he went back down to the boat to retrieve our sleeping bags and a cooler filled with Longero—my favorite Finnish alcohol that's like a grapefruit and gin soda—and Lapin Kulta for him. We ate until we were stuffed and drank until we were delirious. To add a little inner warmth, he used two sticks to grab a golf ball–sized rock from the fire and dropped it into the plastic bottle. We watched as the water instantly boiled. Then he added berries and pine needles, and we sipped what we called pine berry tea. Warmed from the inside out, we cuddled up in our shelter and fell asleep. Two hours later I awoke cold and shaking. The fire had gone out and it was pitch-black. I could feel bits of dirt dropping from the moss and swore I was being attacked by spiders. Thinking I was going to die from the cold, the romance of it all was far from my memory as I shook him awake to relight the fire. We decided to sleep in shifts, tending to the fire for the rest of the night. The next morning he surprised me with a baggie of instant coffee that he added to the plastic bottle (the glass bottle was reserved for drinking water) and did the same boiling rock trick. I was in heaven once again, and we decided to stay and "survive" for two more nights.

Would I have liked champagne, a chocolate cake, maybe a gift that made me feel beautiful and sexy? Absolutely. Was the yacht trip mind-blowingly amazing? You're kidding me, right? Mind officially blown. But, despite the dire lack of trappings on the island in Finland, it was an extraordinary experience, one of my most treasured in life. Because on the island nothing else mattered. We weren't marred by the drama of "real" life. We didn't have the pressures of perfection. We were able to just be ourselves—together.

* * *

It's said that you can't judge a book by its cover, and that's very true. Stop judging people based on their looks, and instead uncover the stories beneath that make them who they are. Your life experiences make you interesting. They also give you something to talk about. When framed and used strategically, they have the ability to illuminate certain sides of you, create an opportunity for deep and revealing conversations, and even help to gain insight from the person you are talking to—extracting substantive information including who he is, what his core values are, and whether you two could possibly be right for each other.

Much more than the art of conversation, framing your stories is an essential component of the formula to get a guy to fall for you hard and fast. It will also help you to get a sense of your date. After you share a story, he will share one of his—I'll show you mine, then you show me yours.

What is love and chemistry, after all? A lot of it is the trust, comfort, and safety in connecting on a deep level as well as the understanding and admiration of who we are at our core, what our beliefs are, our strengths, our vulnerabilities, the adversity that we have overcome and the strength that we were able to derive from it—all that adds up to who we are as individuals and the little things that make us unique and therefore lovable.

How do you show those things about yourself and learn those things about someone else? It can take months, even years, as you slowly peel back the onion, only revealing a little bit more as trust is earned. Or it can take a few strategic conversations of telling your stories. Not to worry, this isn't about oversharing, vomiting your issues, or lying vulnerable and naked on a tabletop. Frame your stories before you tell them so that you know how much you are willing to share, how deep you are open to going, and the purpose of each detail revealed. It might seem as though you're completely exposed. But you're not. It's a false bottom. There is so much more below the depth that you have chosen to show. It's *that* layer of depth that is earned. Here's the awesome thing: because you are seemingly offering up so much, you can then ask questions that prompt him to share something similarly substantive, something that makes him feel, and soon he is exposing who he truly is. You have now tapped into his heart, spirit, and soul, and he will begin to form a bond with you because of the sheer fact that you know so much about him and because he felt something—he felt open. The foundation and environment of trust is being created. To feel love, your heart has to be opened. To open your heart, you have to feel emotions. Telling stories from your core triggers you to feel while simultaneously sharing who you are. But here's the thing—you truly have to tell stories that tap into your core. If you simply listen to his stories, if you act like a sounding board, if you only super-ficially share, he will likely start to feel for you, but you won't feel for him back. Why? Because his heart was tapped and yours was not. This is why some relationships end up being emotionally uneven at an early stage—one person opened, shared, felt, and started to feel, but the other person didn't reciprocate. If you want to feel love from and for another, you have to decide to first trigger yourself to feel. You will feel through sharing. Framing your core stories is the best and most direct heart-tapping path.

But those are the deep-level benefits. Let's talk about why framing your stories is great in the moment.

- Your stories give you something to talk about when you're on a date.

- They illuminate to yourself just how interesting you are (which is essential when it comes to confidence building).

- They help you to show and tell what your core values are.

- They show him that you are coming to the table as a whole, evolved, interesting, and layered person.

WHAT ARE YOUR STORIES?

Look at your core values. The goal is to come up with three stories that illustrate each value. Yes—a total of twenty-one stories! Don't worry, once you start going through your memories, you will flood your mind with more and more experiences. What will be more difficult is organizing them into each core value bucket, then strategically framing them and choosing which couple of details you will highlight to bring the story to life in his mind. Think about your life experiences. What interests and activities and lessons can you share? Once you come up with your stories, it's time to frame them. The way you frame your stories makes a huge difference on their impact and how they are received. That's not to say that you should stay away from stories with substance. Actually the opposite! Dig into them. Expose sides of yourself that might still be raw. Yes, it's time to express vulnerability. Talk about experiences that shaped you. But divulge those stories with purpose—to tell and show who you are and how you came to be, through exposing your choices, mistakes, hardships, interests, and hobbies, plus the reasons, lessons, and understandings that surround them. And . . . know your audience. Once you have your stories, write them down exactly as you would tell them so that they are always present in the back of your mind when you need something to pull out.

Remember, this isn't a novel; it's a story. A short story. Here are a few key elements of purpose-driven storytelling:

Maintain the U structure. The last thing you want to do is drone on and on about something depressing, sickening, harsh, or saddening. You're on a date! You are supposed to have fun. Still, telling a substantive story that reveals some of your vulnerabilities, insecurities, weaknesses, or low points can tend to drop into not-so-upbeat topics. They also make you relatable, triggering the "me too" connection. The key is to only go down for a moment, then swing your story right back up as you tell how that low taught you so much and now you are a better, stronger, more evolved person because of it. Here is why: if you want him to see that you were able to overcome adversity, you have to give a taste of that adversity— but not a mouthful.

Keep it short. Your story should take you less than five minutes to tell. You don't want to lose his attention or make him feel like he never got a word in. Remember: guys like to talk about themselves too. This is an opportunity for back-and-forth sharing. It's a conversation, not a monologue.

Keep it on-purpose. Remember your intention behind the story. Don't ramble or get sidetracked. This is why framing it, writing it down, and practicing it first is a really good idea.

Keep it interesting. Design it as an interesting story with a beginning, middle, and end.

Keep it focused on you. Even if it's a story about your mom thinking she's about to die in New York City, keep it focused on the fact that *you* went to rescue her, you nurtured her, you are the go-to in the family, you are responsible, you don't freak out when faced with challenging moments. This is about you, not your mom. He is investing in you, not your mom. Honestly, at this point he doesn't care about your mom. It's your response that matters.

Be big. Don't just tell stories about minutia. Tell your most interesting, surprising, revealing, shocking, emotionally engaging stories. You won't be telling a story about how you take your dog on a walk every morning and she loves to smell this one particular pink rose. Sure, it's tender and that might be interesting for some people, but probably not to a guy who you are going out with for the first time.

Don't stick to safe subjects, but don't offend either. If you pick up that he shares your political or religious beliefs and you want to talk about it, go right ahead. But dip your toe in the water before jumping in. Don't cannonball into pools of touchy subjects that tend to be polarizing. If you go into gay rights and you have no idea that his brother is openly out, you could be making uneducated statements that shut him down emotionally without you even knowing what you did to mess this one up. Flap your lips about abortion, and you didn't know that his last girlfriend had one and it was excruciatingly emotional for both of them and caused the end of their relationship, and you might be exposing a very sore subject.

Use specific details to paint pictures. Highlight two or three of the most interesting elements. When I say "interesting," I mean the details that *he* will find interesting. So you won't go in depth about the adorable pink bows. But you might go into the five-inch rattle on the rattlesnake or the fact that you were wearing a bikini in the snow. Paint pictures. The most interesting stories make you feel like you can see them unfolding, almost like you were there experiencing them. A picture may be worth a thousand words, but words that paint picture are a part of compelling storytelling.

Be enthusiastic. It's not just the story that's interesting, it's the delivery. Does a head in a talking box with zero voice inflections and little movement make you want to listen? Probably not. Allow your voice to get a little singsongy. Accentuate interesting components with an elevated or exaggerated tone, tempo, or volume. Use your hands. Use a combination of an awesome story, voice changes, and gestures to attract and keep his undivided attention. Remember, this is all still new. He really doesn't have that much invested in you, so you need to keep him interested and pull him in. Then keep him there.

Create opportunities for tangential conversations. If your story involves family, skiing, and New Year's Eve, you have created three tangential conversation opportunities. Even though your focus is family, the topic of skiing might resonate more with him. But after you share your story ask leading questions that help him to go as deeply as you just dove.

Engage him. Don't just talk, talk, talk about yourself. Ask questions. Pick up on the little things that he says, the brushstroke statements or the teeny reveals, and dig a little deeper with them. If he mentions that he isn't really close with his mom anymore and because of that he usually spends the holidays with friends and they throw this awesome party where they all pitch in to cook a deep-fried turkey . . . talk about that tradition, but then pick up on the mom comment. "Why aren't you really close with your mom anymore?" or "You mentioned that you and your mom aren't really close. Do you have a relationship with your dad/siblings/other family members?" Ask questions that engage him, then let him talk as you listen.

CHAPTER 3

How to Get Him

You know after a long day on your feet when you finally settle into bed and your muscles ache as they attempt to let go and succumb to relaxation? Sometimes they hurt so badly that you almost consider getting back up, but you know that if you just surrender for a few minutes, you will get over that uncomfortable feeling and find bliss on the other side. Same goes for some of the things I am going to ask you to do. You will feel awkward at times. You might even hate me for making you feel like a fool, which you're not, by the way. It's just that you are doing something that's different for you. I'm asking you to let go, try something new, and trust that you will get through it and come out a better, more evolved person on the other side. Oh, and with an amazing guy. This is how you are going to get him. . . .

MUST-HAVE FEMININE TRAITS TO CATCH AND KEEP A GREAT MAN

Is he a butt or a boobs guy? Does he find blondes, redheads, or brunettes most beautiful? If he had to choose between an introvert or an extrovert, what would be his preference? When it comes down to it, what do you think is the most attractive thing to a man? The thing that makes him want to attach himself to you and never let go?

What if I told you that none of the above really matters? Sure, beautiful cleavage, a perky butt, silky hair in his favorite color, or a life-of-the-party type of girl might initially draw a guy in, but it's not going to keep him. Surprisingly (or not), men are looking for deeper, more substantive, and enduring traits that for some reason too many women decide not to display—at least not early on in dating and sometimes too little too late. Honestly, if you hide the substantive, authentic, even vulnerable sides of you...you're boring. You're forgettable. Believe me—your surface traits are common. If you want to stand out in the overcrowded dating pool, be you! Plus, highlight these seven traits that turn a guy on more than T&A ever will:

1. Fun and happiness

2. Confidence

3. Independence (also called: A Life)

4. Strength and integrity

5. Vulnerability and openness

6. Femininity and nurturing

7. X Appeal (part of the icing on the cake)

Let me break it down for you.

Are you a happy person? Are you happy with your life, your work, your purpose, your state of being? Or are you that incessant Debbie Downer (sorry, Debbie) who counters a compliment with a "yeah but," who makes snarky comments about smiling couples, who is quick with a complaint and expects to be disappointed? A guy isn't going to make you happy. That's not his job. Nor do you want it to be. A woman who is happy and shows it is highly desirable for a man, because at the end of the day, a guy wants to feel good. He wants to be happy, to laugh, to have fun. He wants to be able to sit next to you watching TV or lie there with you at night and just be. Be happy. He wants to feel enlivened by your smile, refueled by your belief in him, and at peace in your presence.

He also wants to have fun with you! Fun comes from having a spirit that is effervescent, exuberant, enthusiastic, playful, youthful, unjaded, and happy. Don't confuse that with stupid, obnoxious, airheaded, undependable, immature, or even young. Life and work can be so stressful! Your partner is the one person you can let your guard down around. At home or out, when no one else is watching, that's when it's safe to do ridiculous dances, speak in strange voices, just be you—not the "appropriate," contrived, careful-what-you-say-and-do side that you exhibit in the office or even around friends. If you want him to feel like he can have fun with you, you need to not be afraid to have fun with him, even if you look ridiculous.

CONFIDENCE

A confident woman knows her worth. She takes pride in herself, which is apparent through her attitude and appearance. She isn't looking for approval from guys. She knows she's pretty great. She also knows that the right guy will be very lucky to be with her because she has the ability to make him happier than any other woman can. But she's not a bitch about it. And here's the thing: you make him feel that way too—that he can make you happier than any other man can.

Fact is, guys want to feel like they won the prize, like they are dating the head of the cheerleading team. He wants to feel like he's the luckiest guy in the room. Just as he wants you to be proud of him, he wants to be proud of you. If you have a bummer, insecure, self-deprecating, "I'm not so great" attitude, why would he feel like he scored? Whether it's your looks, brain, triumphs, the respect you garner, your career, or simply how you push yourself through pain and get out of your box, he wants to feel like he can show you off. He needs to know that he can confidently bring you home to mom, introduce you to his friends, and accompany him to business dinners with his boss—because you make him look good . . . And you know it.

INDEPENDENCE (ALSO CALLED: A LIFE)

You're busy, driven, self-sufficient, and autonomous. You have your own interests. You're interesting. You're passionate. You have things going on that contribute to high-quality conversations. You have a life! And you love it. You challenge him, but you're not a challenge. You are your best self, raising the bar and inspiring him to be his best self too. Whether it's your business that you adore, or you have emotionally and creatively fulfilling hobbies, the point is that you don't *need* him to fill a void or make you happy. But you *want* him. Translation: you aren't needy. You're already a complete and satisfied person without him. Still, although you may be busy and you can certainly take care of yourself, don't play hard to get or be too difficult to nail down for a date. You still need to show your enthusiasm for him. Be excited to see him. A man wants to feel wanted and special. Just like you do. So when you see him, be totally present. Smile. And be your fabulous and interesting self.

STRENGTH AND INTEGRITY

Can you stand tall when he experiences moments of weakness? Or will you wither and collapse without having his strength? Can you take care of business and hold your own if need be? That strength takes some of the pressure off him and allows him to want to be strong for you, as opposed to making him feel like he *has* to be strong for you.

But, more than the ability to take care of business when times get tough, are you strong in your values and beliefs? Or do you waver, fluctuate, appear wishy-washy or easily influenced? Do you feel the need to consult friends, family, chat rooms, or Internet hangouts in order to make decisions? Do you come to conclusions by committee or collective consensus, or are you confident enough to make up your own mind? Who are you? What do you believe in? Do you stand by it? Do you have integrity? Can he depend on what you say? Do your actions align with your words? Or are your words and beliefs worthless? A woman who has unshakable beliefs, who shows and tells the same story, makes a man feel safe. A feeling of safety is one of the most crucial elements when it comes to a man's ability to trust, let his guard down, and open his heart completely. He knows that he can depend on you for good or for bad, in sickness and in health, weakness and triumph. In moments of uncertainty, the one thing that he can be certain of is you—because you are certain of you.

VULNERABLITY AND OPENNESS

I'm not talking about being a withering flower, a damsel in distress, or a gaping wound. Vulnerability is true strength. It is confidence. It is "Here I am." Vulnerability is the ultimate connector. It is the seed of love, friendship, empathy, and innovation. Being vulnerable is about being real, open, and not shut down. Exposing your weaknesses may seem to be the opposite of strength, but real strength is shown in your ability to express your fragility, your pain points, your insecurities, and even revealing things that you have done that you are not proud of or regret, without fear of judgment. Real strength is confident vulnerability.

Show him that he makes you feel vulnerable—in a good way. The best way—because your heart is open. Show him how much you love him. Tell him how crazy you are about him. Let him know that you have never felt this way before. When you are open and vulnerable with him, you're also showing him that you trust him. Trust, both trusting and being trusted, is one of the most important things for a man. By being closed off, you are showing him that you don't trust him with your heart, you don't trust him with your body, you don't trust him with you. You don't trust that he can take care of you, provide for you, support you. By opening up to him, you are saying, "I trust you with me." Your emotional vulnerability makes him feel more confident about your feelings for him and therefore allows him to be emotionally vulnerable and open about his for you. Within that place of vulnerability, you will connect on a deeper, more substantive level than ever before.

FEMININITY AND NURTURING

Men feel even more masculine when they are with a feminine woman—and that in and of itself turns a man on! Femininity is about both appearance and attitude. Being feminine is about embracing your beauty, softness, tenderness, nurturing, the sweet side that men just don't generally have. Be a woman! Be a girly girl! Wear dresses and lipstick and smell good. I'm not suggesting that you submit, succumb, or hand over your power—who says you can't be powerful in a dress and stilettos?! Enjoy making yourself look good. You just might notice that you feel good too.

Be nurturing. One of the feminine traits that a man isn't often imbued with is the natural instinct to nurture. Because it's lacking in them, they often crave it in us. You can be vulnerable and show him that you need him, but you also can take care of him. No matter how strong, independent, and masculine he is, all men love to be nurtured, taken care of, and even babied at times. Showing him that you can be a nurturer lets him know that he can drop his guard around you and that it's okay and safe to need you. When a guy exposes weakness, when he lets you in to see his vulnerable side, that's where your power lies—not in a way that's game playing or manipulative but to create an enduring relationship based on feeling safe and at home with you, just like his mother used to do.

X APPEAL: THE ALLURING, CAPTIVATING, AND INTOXICATING TRAIT THAT MOST WOMEN LACK

I'm sure you have experienced it too: he's such a great guy, but there is just *some*thing missing. What is that *some*thing? That missing *some*thing is the reason that some of the most "perfect" women who seem like they have it all—a beautiful face, amazing body, successful career, interesting life experiences, etc., etc. . . . can't keep a guy beyond date four, or even date two, and they don't know why. They are missing the X Appeal.

So what's the X Appeal? It's the total package (above) wrapped up in an alluring, enticing, and captivating bow. It's the essential icing on the cake. It's the magic sauce that transforms a dish from great to addictive. It's that intoxicating scent and lingering feeling that doesn't seem to fade but instead leaves you wanting more. There are seven traits that contribute to the X Appeal, including:

1. Purpose and core values: knowing who you are

2. Being interesting and interested

3. Femininity: in body language, verbal communication, energy

4. Effort: outward appearance

5. Attitude: "that chick" abundance, radiance, confidence, sexy and you know it

6. Flirt-ability

7. Intrigue: magnetic pull, playful, challenge, memorable

Yes, it seems like a lot. And it is. It's a lot of little nuanced details that when woven together create the X Appeal. But, for starters, it's much of what I reveal in the "How to Walk into a Room and Own It" and "How to Flirt" sections below, so make sure to study and practice them. (For added guidance on X Appeal, visit ScrewingTheRules.com/Products.)

HOW TO WALK INTO A ROOM AND OWN IT

When I was young, I was always the girl who was cute, not pretty; sweet, not sexy; a friend, not a girlfriend; a follower, but never, ever a popular girl. I wanted to be one of the "cool" girls who sauntered around school flaunting her stuff. But late bloomer that I was, I had nothing to flaunt. Because it was assigned to me (and incessantly reinforced), I owned the sweet, innocent, friend/follower role, along with the insecurities that came with it: a distinct lack of sexual self-assuredness and the inability to express myself in a sensual way for fear of feeling and, even more so, looking stupid. Thankfully, my sexuality began to blossom, and I slowly transitioned into girlfriend material as opposed to the "good friend." But, as a result of my stunted start, I had to force myself to learn how to strut my stuff without hearing that voice in my head telling me that I indeed looked as stupid as I felt.

Because I was armed with the ability to be an observer (thanks to years of being ignored), I began to watch the dance between men and women, and I learned to emulate, then improve upon, the tactics that enticed the opposite sex to take notice. Once my carefully crafted mating call was conceived, I put it into action to see whether it was possible to perfect the approach and be the girl who walked into a room and owned it.

* * *

Have you ever watched one those women who seems to have it all? She lights up a room when she enters it, simultaneously warming and enlivening it with her presence. And, despite the fact that everyone angles his or her head to take in her presence, she doesn't seem to notice. Yet somehow she notices everyone as she makes each person who is graced by her eye contact feel important.

Do you want to be that chick? Next time one enters a room that you're in, watch her. Really take her in. Notice how she moves her body, what her facial expressions say, how she styles her hair and clothes. What is it about her that's so intoxicating? It's not just looks. In fact, if two women walk into a room at the same time—one is stunning but insecure with her eyes to the ground and a frown on her face, and the other is okay-looking but she is radiant with this knowing smile and a certain air about her, people might note the pretty girl first, but that attention will quickly shift to the woman who's presence is beautiful from the inside out.

There is something about confidence that is sexier than high cheekbones, a pair of Dior stilettos, a cleavage-baring camisole, or even a slit so high that your whole thigh is exposed in that Angelina Jolie way. It's time for you to embody that hot chick hidden inside you. That chick who knows exactly what to say, what to do, and how to walk into a room and own it. She knows how to attract attention, exude a magnetism that you can't resist, and get her way. That chick is the wild, sexual beast lying dormant within you. She knows how to be in control, own a room, hold seductive eye contact, and smile so magnetically that others around can't help but be drawn in. She gives the impression of having complete confidence in herself and her body, and she seriously turns guys on until they can't help but be lured in. Give that chick a pseudonym if you want (but be careful not to let it slip . . . That could get awkward).

It's time to get to know that chick. Sit with her, try to understand her, examine and develop her. And be her! Think about this:

- Who is she?
- What's her name? (You can just call her "that chick" if you want.)
- What does she wear?
- How does she do her hair?
- Does she wear makeup?
- Does she wear high heels?
- What's her attitude?
- What is it about her that makes her so attractive and magnetic?
- What quality of men respond to her?
- How does she talk with women?
- How does she talk with men?
- What does she talk about with men?

Now practice being her. If you never wear high heels and that hot chick does, get some gorgeous stilettos and start strutting your stuff at home alone until you feel comfortable—and beyond that, confident—walking four inches higher. If you never do your hair and don't really care but that chick does, start practicing with sexy but practical styles. Go to a makeup counter at the mall and ask them to teach you how to put on simple but feature-accentuating makeup.

This is about putting some effort into it—into yourself! And therefore into finding your one.

More than the superficial—hair and makeup and sexy clothes—confidence is about attitude. It's a feeling. It's walking into a room and knowing, "I got this." It's smiling and approaching a guy and just saying hi and knowing that he wants to talk to you. Now *that* is sexy!

HOW TO FLIRT

- Be honest. Does flirting make you nervous?

- Do you get quiet, insecure, or awkward when it comes to talking with guys you're potentially interested in?

- Are you sick of feeling like you're making a fool of yourself?

- Or maybe you just wonder what you're doing wrong?

- Did you know that flirting isn't just about the initial conversation, but it can also make or break a date?

Dating doesn't have to suck. In fact, it can be fun! You just have to get out of your rigid, insecure, awkward, or over-the-top way and learn a few strategies that will help you not only get comfortable with and master the art of the flirt but have fun with it!

Flirting is a strategy, but it feels like a spell. And that's where the power is. At its most basic level, flirting is composed of three key elements, weaving together attitude, body language, and conversation like a fluid dance. And although you definitely want to make *him* feel amazing, there is one secret that you must know in order to pull it off: *you are in control the entire time.*

Once you get the strategy down, then you fill it in with the fun. And that's where you really have to dig deep (and why you did all that work in the previous sections). Flirting isn't just about the T&A; it's about tactic.

There is an art to the flirt, a dance, a rhythm. You don't want to come across as too coy or too trashy. You don't want to come across as too submissive or too abrasive. You want to dance along the center in a controlled yet effervescent manner that makes you look sexy and makes him feel sexy. If you know how to work your magic, you can reel in almost any guy in mere minutes. But it's a juggling act, one that combines the eyes, body, lips, voice, hands, and words. It's also individualized, playing to your personal strengths and shading your weaknesses. Flirting well takes practice, but more than anything it takes confidence—true or faked. Either one, honestly, is fine. Even if you're faking it at first, once you get the hang of it you'll be a natural.

The most successful flirts do more than draw him in; they make him feel like the luckiest, most interesting man in the world—or at least in the room and in that moment. Now it's your turn to learn how to harness this incredible power. Let's start with the three phases of the U Flirt Strategy:

1. Be radiant.

2. Be vulnerable.

3. Be honeyed.

Again, with the U Strategies you are starting high, going down deep, then popping back up. What I mean is this:

BE RADIANT

You are confident without being cocky or confrontational, warm without being sleepy or motherly, and effervescent without being bubbly or airy. You are in control but a little coy about it. You are magnetic in your body language, energy, and words. You make him want to rise to the occasion without making him feel like it's an impossible feat. You are witty but not sarcastic and definitely not a bitch. Your radiance is the lasso that you have now successfully secured around his neck. Now all you have to do is pull him in—and that requires a dose of vulnerability.

BE VULNERABLE

This is the low point of the "U." It's where you aren't on, but instead you're you. It's the scariest, but often most captivating, component. It takes strength to show weakness. It takes confidence to expose vulnerability. Being vulnerable creates an environment of trust. And feeling trusted is one of the most important things to a man. It's also what endears him to you, softens his heart, and compels him to notice that you're different from all of the other façades walking around—and that makes him want to know more. While I definitely don't want you to unload your drama, become a crying mess, or expose your insecurities upon first meeting the guy, you should let your guard down a little and show a flash of what's hiding under the mask. You're letting him in on a secret, which makes him feel special. It's those images of your reality that will intrigue and excite him about you. Be real. Reveal little bits of your authentic self through your conversations—the framed stories that illuminate your core values and simultaneously show just how interesting you are. It's those glimpses of your depth, of your quirks and your layers, that will implant you in his mind long after you have left his personal space. Now that he's in, boost him up and make him feel like a god (believe me, guys eat this shit up).

BE HONEYED

Though an uncommon word, with its layered meaning and lingering experience, "honeyed" perfectly depicts the next phase of the U Flirt Strategy. Sweet, flattering, enticing, seductive, and luscious—you're basically making the guy feel great! You are boosting his ego without overindulging him. But that's okay, because you built yourself up in Phase 1, reeled him into you in Phase 2, and now you're saying, "And I think you're pretty great too" in Phase 3. Here's how:

1. Build him up
2. Challenge him
3. Compliment him

Here's an example:

BUILD HIM UP

"Wow, that was a strong handshake! I bet you give amazing massages."

CHALLENGE HIM

"Though I don't know that you can get deep enough for me. I love seriously strong and deep massages. I'll let you massage my shoulders for a minute so I can see if you can really get in there and relax me. I have been so stressed lately."

COMPLIMENT HIM

"I have to say, I'm impressed. My massage therapist would be jealous if I told him what great hands you have."

Why does this work? You made him feel good. Then you challenged him, questioning his worth and making him want to prove himself to you. Once he has a goal of making you happy, he is invested in you. Then back up the side of the "U" as you tell him that you're impressed, stroking his ego a little bit.

The order of the U Flirt Strategy is key. Skip to Phase 3 and flatter him first, and you're just like every other girl out there. What makes you unique? Your high-value worth. Show him that! Make him want to work for it. Make him want to impress you. Part of his impressing you is helping you. A man likes to feel trusted—and useful. If you show him your vulnerable side, he won't be able to help himself in wanting to fix something by being protective of you or offering solutions. And because you showed that you trust him and created a safe environment for vulnerability, he will be more compelled to share something about himself, too. And now he has invested in you. Finally, as a reward for his good behavior (have I mentioned that men are like dogs and that's a really good thing?)—Phase 3: build him up and tell him how great he is!

This U Flirt Strategy is great on the first few dates too, obviously because you should be flirting!

Throughout the entire "U," you have to show and tell, another three-element strategy, but this one isn't in phases. You will be weaving all three together like a fluid dance.

1. Attitude

2. Body language

3. Conversation

ATTITUDE: YOU'RE ON!

From the moment you step out of your car door, you are on. Imagine that you are on a reality television show being followed by a film crew. You open your car door upon arriving at the restaurant, bar, party, or even just to the grocery store or gym, and those cameras are on you. Act like it! You can no longer think, "It's okay to look sloppy, no one is watching me." Now they are watching. In fact, they always were; you just didn't realize it. You may have missed hundreds of opportunities to be picked up on by the love of your life because you were in the headspace of "I don't care, no one is watching." You may have chosen to make yourself invisible by wearing an old and ugly grey sweat suit, your hair in a rat's nest mess atop your head, and a scowl on your face, and you're right—no one saw you. Their eyes passed right over you, including the eyes of the guy you should be cuddling with right now. But that's okay. You'll get another chance. Just don't allow for another missed opportunity.

Your attitude is of radiance! You're hot and you know it. Own it! Eat it, swallow it, be it. Flip that light switch on and step out of your car with that hot chick attitude oozing from your core—that you discovered in the last section! You are on-purpose and ready to see and be seen. Be that hot chick *now*.

Once you find the guy who you want to dedicate some of your super-powered attention to, don't act like you're too good. Do the opposite. Whenever you are placing your attention on him, make him feel amazing!

MAKE HIM FEEL AMAZING!

One of the main areas of importance when it comes to flirting is making your prey (for lack of a better word) feel like a total stud. And remember, just because it's how guys are wired, when he first sees you he's thinking about how you will be in bed. You don't want to come across as a spaz, a bore, or an attention whore. You want to come across as fun, light, passionate, maybe slightly wild, interesting, experienced (but not too experienced), and able to let go. Here's how:

Smile just a little bit, then momentarily stare (not glare, stare). Smile softly with both your eyes and your mouth. Before it gets awkward, look away and jump right back into what you were doing or the conversation you were having before you just couldn't help yourself but stare for a moment too long at him.

Say hi! You don't have to wait for him to come and talk to you. Don't be shy; you can go over and say hello.

Don't be plain vanilla. Not that there is anything wrong with vanilla (I love it when it comes to ice cream), but, when it comes to asserting your personality, show your sprinkles, cherries, swirl, chips, and nuts. When talking to him, show passion and joie de vivre. Don't give him your bio or resume; instead, tell him who you are and what you have seen, and weave a few fascinating life experiences into the conversation. This isn't just about him. You have done and seen some pretty cool things, too. Let him know how honestly interesting you are.

Be interested and interesting. You are engaged in his stories and what he has to say, and you tell him stories that are animated and unique so that he is equally engrossed in what you have to say.

Don't be a Debbie Downer. Even if you're having a low day, your life doesn't suck in general. Bring out the positive. No one wants to be brought down by talking to you. Now is not the time to vent about what a horrible day you had or how much you hate your job. Be positive. I'm not saying to fake it and be someone you're not, but be someone that he enjoys talking to, someone who brightens his evening, makes him feel good, and he'll remember that time talking to you with a smile on his face.

He is the most important thing in that moment. Do *not* do the look over his shoulder glance to see whether someone else might be of more appealing. Hone in, focus, listen, engage, touch his arm on occasion, be totally present in that moment.

Simultaneously, do *not* be overly into him, aggressive, or obnoxious, and don't make a scene. Maintain control.

You want to be sexy yet comfortable, in control yet relaxed, interesting and deep yet effervescent and fun, confident yet interested, aware and present yet not a puppy affixed to his leg, and you are on yet not always angling for attention. Now that you have the attitude down, here's how to embody it. . . .

BODY LANGUAGE

More than what and how much you say, a picture can be worth a thousand words—the same goes for your body language. From the moment he sees you, your first impression is being made, even if it's from across a room with no actual interaction. As I already said, when you are out, be aware that you are being watched. You are on—because you don't know where you are going to meet your next boyfriend or maybe even your one! What if you miss out because your body language communicated for you before you even got a chance to say hi?

Guys can sense insecurity. Especially when you are oozing it through body language. What does your body language express?

- Fine? **F**reaked out, **i**nsecure, **n**ervous, **e**motional?
- Shut down?
- Expecting rejection? Already rejected.
- Skeptical or not trusting? Jaded.
- Desperate and needy? Please like me.
- You can't hurt me! I'm a successful and intimidating woman!
- . . . Or confident, sexy, sassy, fun, and alluring?

If you want to be seen as confident, sexy, sassy, fun, and alluring, imagine and attempt to embody:

- Jennifer Lopez
- Kim Kardashian
- Rihanna
- Marilyn Monroe
- Sharon Stone
- Scarlett Johansson
- Cleopatra
- Jessica Rabbit
- Betty Boop

Here are a few tips to help.

Make and keep eye contact. Stare for one second too long. Not a creepy glare, but a stare, with a slight smile and a knowing twinkle in your eye.

U Flirt Eyes Strategy. The U Flirt Strategy isn't just about the words you say; it's the thoughts you convey with your eyes. A woman's eyes can be very expressive once she understands how to use them. When you look at a guy you think might have potential, practice the U Flirt Strategy in your mind and project it through your eyes. Here's how: Look him up and down as you think, "This guy has potential." Then question his potential and wonder whether he really has anything to offer that will be enough to keep your interest. You're not sure. Finally, pick a feature or characteristic that pulls you in—it can be his authentic smile, his laugh, his kind eyes, his confidence, etc. Yeah, he just might have what it takes to make you want more.

That entire U thought process occurs within the few seconds that you're looking at him, making sure that you've already hooked him with eye contact. When done well, he will read your U thoughts, challenging him to want to impress you and prove his worth to you.

Present with your posture! Roll your shoulders back (which is different from the overt act of simply sticking your chest out). Allow for a slight arch in your back—it's sexy and pops your butt while freeing your hips for movement.

Two o'clock shoulders, eleven o'clock face. While standing with your chest, shoulders, and face directly in front of him works in the business world, communicating your confidence and letting him know that you are just as competent as he is, the stance is too aggressive and masculine in the dating realm. This isn't a showdown. You are flirting. Adjust your body placement accordingly. If he is standing at twelve o'clock, your front shoulder should be angled at two o'clock, with your back shoulder at eight o'clock. Angle your face just slightly less away at eleven o'clock. The stance isn't completely open, but it also isn't closed off. It's alluring. It says that you have something inside that you are protecting. You want to draw and lure him in.

Secret Smile. Smile. It's sexy. Just make it a secret, or sideways, smile. Yes, we are keeping with the off-center theme. Let him see half of your smile, showing him that you have a secret and that he wants to know what it is. A side smile is a little mischievous, creating wonderment and allure. Sometimes you can give him the full face. But that's a gift. A big toothy grin can appear desperate, childish, or crazy—none of which are sexy.

Lift your chin. The goal isn't to look stuck up or snobby. Just confident.

Relax your arms. Loosen up and let your arms fall at your sides and be open to receive. You definitely don't want to cross your arms or have your hands on your hips—that looks too authoritative and masculine.

Take a beat. Imagine that hot, cocky guy at a party who sits back on the sofa and takes in the sights. He has women lining up to talk to him. He isn't a jerk. He's smiling in a way that makes you need to know what's on his mind. But he's deliberate in his movements and his attitude. That's how you want to feel.

A little touch. The occasional little touch on his wrist or even his side abs (if you're standing) is okay. It shows that you aren't rigid and you are interested, and it makes him imagine you touching him more. But don't touch too much. You want him to work to get more where that came from.

Play, push, and pull. Lean in a little, then lower your tone and slightly pull back as you imagine pulling his energy into yours.

Mirroring. Mirrored body language is a sign of connection. Don't do it obsessively, but do move your body into the same relaxed position as his and show him how in sync you are.

Slow down. Take your time with your movements. Be deliberate. Every move you make matters and expresses something about you. If you are trying to do everything at once, you will be seen as manic.

Stop nodding. When you shake your head up and down repeatedly and over and over again as someone is talking, even if you are in authentic agreement, it appears fake and makes him feel like he needs to spit out what he's saying faster.

Play with your hair. There is a difference between twirling your hair like a child and delicately fingering your hair in a sexy way that makes him imagine his hands following the same path.

Monkey see, monkey follow. Occasionally use your hands to lead his eyes along your skin. Place your hands on your neck and his eyes will follow. Slide up to your lips and he's right there with you.

Don't motor. You know when someone is quickly bouncing their foot or leg up and down so fast that it feels like the floor is vibrating? That's motoring. It shows that you are nervous and creates unease—and often disinterest—in the person you are speaking to. If you are a natural motorer, take a beat, exhale, and stop.

Don't be a talking head. That's boring. Show that you have energy, enthusiasm, and life by using your hands when you speak to help enhance the conversation. Emoting with your hands, arms, and body is sexy, because it makes guys think about your body and its movements. It also shows that you are physically expressive, which is equally sexy.

Seated? The above still apply. Plus:

- Let your arms comfortably rest on the sides of the chair or on the bar or table.

- Cross your legs loosely above your knees and let your feet angle apart.

Your Walk. It says a lot about you. It's an instant giveaway when it comes to your personality and confidence. Your walk should always be purpose driven, deliberate, and slowed down. Relax your body, allowing your arms to move freely at your sides and your hips to hinge back and forth. Keep your shoulders rolled back, your chin confident, and a sly little secret smile on your face. As you walk, make deliberate eye contact with several people as you pass. Let them see that you see them. When you make eye contact, expand your smile just a touch more so that they feel like they are just a little bit more special than everyone else. Then refresh your gaze back to your purpose (wherever you are going).

CONVERSATION

What you say, what you choose not to say, and how you say it has the power to deepen your relationships or make them superficial. An interesting conversation can instantly captivate a man and make him want to know more. Here are the basics:

Pull him in with your voice! In business we tend to push our speech. You are speaking *at* someone. Your tone is forceful so that you can get your point across. In dating, you want to do more pulling. Pull him into you instead of pushing yourself into him. Slow your tempo, drop your tone, even quiet your voice just a touch. Soften the edges and the harshness as you add a little molasses to your voice. Allow your speech to come from your stomach instead of your throat, and pull him into your depths. Imagine that he is sitting in a chair. Pull your voice and he is at the edge of his seat. Push your voice and you are pushing him into the back of his chair, making him feel cornered and therefore defensive or shut down.

Don't be monotonous. A monotone voice is like flat-lining the conversation. You will sound more like a bored professor giving a lecture and lose his interest very quickly. Speaking in a more sing-songy way keeps his attention on you.

Don't be afraid to challenge him a little. Verbally spar with him if you feel he's up for it and if you can maintain your ground.

Take a beat. When he says something, it's okay to take a beat before you respond. Remember—be deliberate. What you say matters. You can still be witty and charming and verbally joust a bit. But have confidence in what you say. Taking a beat helps you to refocus and pushes your speech from a confident place.

Show off a little! If you have particular knowledge about a topic he brings up, give him just a taste of your insight, showing him that you have something to offer, without making him feel like he is being schooled. Know about wine, music, or food? Throw in a couple of facts and insight. You are so much more than just a random chick, you have something to bring to the table. Let him know that.

It's all in the details. Don't be brief, but remember the details. Pick out a few that are particularly interesting. That's where your stories get good, and that's how they are remembered.

Uh, like, you know, anyway, in fact. Those are all filler words. Avoid them. When used too often they make you sound stupid, childish, insecure, uninterested, and one-upping or too good—in that order.

Don't giggle. Laughing at funny things—even if it's at yourself—is great! Giggling during inappropriate moments, uncomfortable silences, or just at everything he says makes you appear nervous, insecure, childish, and air-headed.

Smile when you talk. You can tell when someone is smiling on the other end of the phone because their tone and tempo change. Smile! It lights up your face, makes him feel special, and makes what you say sound fun.

Be attentive. Eye contact builds credibility and trust. But beyond looking at the person you are talking to, participate in the conversation. Conversation is give and take. I say something, you respond. You say something, I respond. It's not a pissing match of who has the better story, who can be more interesting, who is better, bigger, more. Engage in the conversation. How? Listen to what he says. Respond to what he says by asking a question or contributing your own thoughts to his. Share personal stories. *Don't* listen to what he says, all the while having something that you want to make sure you get to say. That causes you to be distracted from what he's saying, forcing you to blurt out your point as soon as he finishes his. The problem with that? You aren't engaging. He can tell whether you are paying attention or whether you're just nodding your head and saying, "That's interesting." Engaging doesn't mean that you can repeat everything he just said. Engaging means that you listen, process the content, think, then contribute—in the form of a statement, question, remark, or similar scenario.

Make him feel interesting. Shine the spotlight on him. Yes, let him shine! A man wants to feel interesting. If you make him feel that way, he will then walk away thinking that the conversation was, in fact, very interesting. Even if you were bored to death.

A lot goes into the flirt that needs to be seen (not just read). Watch me go into full flirt mode—plus learn a guy's insight—so you can do it, too. "How to Flirt" is online at ScrewingTheRules.com/Products.

FEMININE COMMUNICATION: PHONE, E-MAIL, TEXT: THE DOS, DON'TS, AND WHAT TO EXPECT

Stop being so polite. Stop being so abrasive. Stop couching. Stop being a bitch. Was that confusing? When it comes to communicating—be it on the phone, by e-mail or text, or in person, there are five key elements that make all the difference:

1. Attitude

2. Word choice

3. Motivation

4. Timing

5. Length

ATTITUDE

Women tend to have a tough time communicating in a direct but feminine way. We fear that asking for what we need is a burden. In an attempt to protect ourselves or the person we are talking with, we overcompensate by using softening or aggressive words, by talking in circles and lists in a way that seems like we are trying to sell or justify our needs. Both create misunderstandings and false impressions. Let me tell you something: your needs are valid. Speak up and be heard. Just do it in an assertive, unapologetic, and direct but sweet and authentic way. And those aren't contradictions. Think about how men communicate. Directly. Now remember that both men and women communicate the way we want to be communicated with. Follow his lead.

Think of a man like a dog. If you speak in a direct, clear, and positive way, you will get the desired effect. You are not demanding but you can be commanding. Have you ever tried to explain something to your dog? You give this whole paragraph as to why you really need her to go outside and pee because you are going out for the night and you really don't want her to pee in the house. And she just stares at you. But if you say in a direct, commanding, but sweet and uplifting way, "Go pee!" she runs outside, does her business, and runs back in with her head lifted and tail wagging, proud of her accomplishment. Of course you then reward her with a treat, reinforcing that she was a good dog, increasing the chance that she will behave in a favorable way next time. Same goes with men.

WORD CHOICE

Could/Can vs. Would/Will

Don't think there's much of a difference? Men do. The words "could" or "can" are viewed as unattached, weak, manipulative, demeaning, noncommittal. "Would" or "will" signal a direct, personal request.

For example:

- You say: "Can you take me to dinner tonight?"
- He hears: "Can you afford to take me to dinner tonight?" or "Are you available to take me to dinner?"

He is taking the word "can" as being literal. Yes, he *can* take you to dinner, but he feels like you aren't giving him a choice in the matter unless he comes up with a great excuse to get out of it. But "*Will* you take me to dinner?" is the actual question you want to ask. "Will" gives him a choice. He doesn't feel trapped by your question. You are also expressing both strength and vulnerability in a direct way by voicing your desire, and that is something that he respects.

In *Men Are from Mars, Women Are from Venus*, John Grey illustrates the would/could difference in a brilliantly basic way: imagine that your boyfriend gets down on one knee, holds up a ring box to you, and with tears in his eyes asks, "Could you marry me?"

Weak. "Yeah, I could," you think, "but I don't know that I want to now."

- You say: "Do you want to go to the movies with me tonight?"

- He hears: "Are you in the mood to go to the movies tonight?"

- How he might answer: "No, I feel like hanging out at home." Or "No, I'm pretty tired tonight." Or simply, "Nah."

- How you might take it: rejection. And then your mind goes on to play tricks on you.

Admit it, you use the words "could," "can," and "want" because you are couching your desires and needs. You don't want to come across as demanding so instead you inadvertently come across as passive-aggressive, manipulative, and detached. Be direct. Ask for what you want. "Will you take me to dinner tonight?"

MOTIVATION

Should vs. Want

"Should" vs. "want" isn't about word choice. It's about what motivates you to offer to do something versus what motivates him. Women often offer to do things for others because we feel like we should, because it's the right thing to do, or because we want to be helpful. More often than not, men offer to do things for others only because they want to. If they didn't want to, they wouldn't offer. If a man offers to do something for you, instead of saying, "No it's okay, I can do it myself" or "Are you sure?" say, "I would love that! Thank you so much." It makes him feel good to do things for you. It makes him feel useful and needed. Reward him by being grateful. And he will do it again. If you don't reward him, he will feel unappreciated, and he is less likely to continue to *want* to do things to please you—and therefore he won't offer.

In the same breath, men aren't mind readers. If he isn't offering, it isn't necessarily because he doesn't want to do it. He just doesn't know what it is that you want him to do. Which goes back to communication must #1—have a direct attitude.

TIMING

Men aren't known for their multitasking abilities. If you want to communicate something to him, have the conversation when he isn't focused on something else. If you accidentally do interrupt him when he is in the midst of something else, be aware that he might not be fully paying attention to what you are saying and as a result might not remember what you said. Or he could get annoyed.

LENGTH

Keep it brief. Don't meander. When you need something, there is no need to explain unless he asks. If you go on and on with the story of why you need it, in his mind you are trying to justify it, making him feel like he has no choice, and there he goes again feeling manipulated.

Now, let's talk about the e-mailing, phoning, and texting.

E-MAIL = INFORMATION COLLECTING

E-mail is the best segue out of online communication or after a quick in-person introduction. More than an opportunity to prequalify through strategic questions (which we will go over in a later section), you can also do additional research to see whether this guy is truly who he says he is and to get more scoop than he reveals. How? His e-mail address! Google it. It could reveal his Facebook page, other chat rooms that he contributes to, or his company's website. Even if he asks for your phone number, do not give it out until you feel comfortable with him through an ample prequalification process.

PHONE = INFORMATION COLLECTING /
CHEMISTRY REVEALING

Having a phone conversation before a first date is a great way to prequalify on another level, as well as to gauge your initial chemistry. He will likely give you his number first, which is great! Because you want to be the one doing the calling. Why? Because you are in control of when you have the conversation. You don't want to be taken off guard, you want to be in the right headspace, and you want to make sure that you have the time to talk so you aren't feeling rushed. When you call him, block your number (by dialing *67 before dialing his number) in case the call doesn't go well. Try to have your first call during a time of day when you don't have other pressing concerns on your plate. At the end of the workday or while driving in your car tend to be great times. Get physically comfortable so that you can be emotionally comfortable to be yourself, be present and engaged, maybe even get raw and be a little vulnerable thanks to the sense of safety that the distance of a phone creates. The phone is where your truths often start coming out because what you say is generally not contrived, planned, or even thought out. You say what's on your mind. You also might go into greater detail and expose unexpected feelings. If it seems right, start telling some of your stories so that you can begin to dig into core values—both yours and his. After the first call you should decide on a date—or not. If he doesn't ask you out while on the call and instead you become phone buddies (or worse—text buddies), you can take it upon yourself to say, "Although I enjoy hearing your voice, I'd love to meet you in the flesh!" Then let him do the final asking, "Let's go out to dinner." If he offers coffee, a movie, or any other date that isn't conducive for real conversation in a comfortable environment that allows you to let your guard down, feel free to say, "I'd love to go out with you. How about a drink or dinner instead so that we can really relax without having to get back to work / have time to unwind a bit / really talk." It's okay to ask for what you want, as long as you stay in the feminine while doing it.

The immediate gratification of texting is best used to let him know that you are thinking about him without having to commit to a ten-minute call, confirm a date without having to interrupt his day, flirt, engage in witty banter, and get to know his off-the-cuff personality. But, as with any form of communication, be aware of how often you text and be sure to take your conversations to the next level so that you don't end up in a text-only relationship. Here are a few things to be aware of.

When to begin texting: When you begin to text for the first time, try to have a date set already. If you exchange numbers and initial texts at first meeting, make sure you soon move the conversation onto a phone call or in-person meeting. It is way too easy to get carried away and exchange sexually driven texts before you ever meet in person. On the other end of the spectrum, texting is often the ruin of a relationship before it even starts. Why? Because you start texting too early and text too often, before you have a foundation built and with no plans to meet in person. And then what happens? He becomes bored and disappears.

Entertainment: You are not his entertainment. And he isn't yours. It's actually one of the most common relationship-killing texting problems. What I mean is this: You text him saying, "Hi." Or, "I'm bored." Or, "What are you up to?" You have nothing interesting to share and no questions to ask so you are reaching out to him to see whether he has anything engaging to say. Not okay. Talking about mundane things over text is not a good idea until you both have invested more into the relationship and have developed true feelings on a substantive foundation. Until that is established, he is not there for your entertainment. He has better things that he is actually currently doing with his day. And you are not there for his, because I certainly hope that you also have better and more interesting things you're doing with yours.

Tone: You think you are being funny, sarcastic, or witty, but you may actually be coming across as rude, bitchy, or crass. Remember that your texts are stripped of tone and facial expression—no matter how many emoticons you include. One way to test your tone is to reverse it and imagine that he is sending the text to you. Say it out loud, minus voice inflections, and decide if it comes across as intended in your mind.

Grammar and spelling: Auto"correct" can create some seriously embarrassing miscommunication. But it's not just autocorrect that needs to be screened before the message is sent. While typing too fast, you might miss words, use incorrect grammar, or spell something wrong, inadvertently making you look careless or like an idiot. And then there are the LOL, OMG, WTF, and TTYL abbreviations that—surprise, surprise—not everyone appreciates. Don't misrepresent yourself due to speed texting. Spell-check!

Think before you send: It's easy to send a quick, thoughtless text as a knee-jerk response to a call, e-mail, thought, or text. Before you slam your fingers into the phone as you give him a piece of your mind, stop and think. Are you going to regret this text in ten minutes? What about tomorrow? If you are fired up and not completely able to control your emotions, take a beat and don't hit send. Instead, again, reverse it. Imagine that he is sending that response to you. How would you take it?

The rule of thumb: Your texts should not be longer than the length of your thumb, especially if the content is emotional. If what you have to say is lengthier, pick up the phone or send an e-mail instead. No one wants to receive text message novels.

Follow his lead: If he sends brief texts, use his length as a template for your text length. If you scroll back and see that you are the one who is wordy and he responds with just one word or a brief sentence, think about how that might be coming across to him. Are your levels of interest and neediness also uneven? Guys communicate with you the way they want to be communicated with.

Timing is everything: You don't want to be the one who is always texting first. That gets annoying. You also don't want to be the one who texts several times for each one of his. That appears needy. Follow his lead when it comes to how often you text.

The sexy factor: It's okay to flirt over text. In fact, it's great! What you don't want to do is get carried away and start creating an image of you that is inaccurate. Will you regret what you send the next day?

Photos: Sending photos is great—even if you haven't yet met in person. Even slightly sexy photos are okay, as long as you don't go over the edge. Particularly with online dating, sending photos makes the other person feel special because you took that photo just for him. Plus, it further affirms that you are a real person and not a catfish.

When to respond: Text is a form of communication meant to provide immediate gratification. Don't play games and wait two days before you respond. That's sending the signal that you aren't truly interested and that you are a game player. Respond when you see his text. That doesn't mean to obsessively check your phone. You have a life, remember? When you see that he texts, send a response. It's just as you would do with a friend. She texts, you respond. Right?

Post-date thank-you: The post-date thank-you is the perfect opportunity to text. You just had a lovely time—either that night or the night before—and you are letting him know that you enjoyed it without invading his space. I go into more detail on this in a later section.

ICEBREAKERS AND CONVERSATION STARTERS

You wouldn't necessarily think of the grocery store as a great place to meet single and looking men. Think again. I was starving after a day of meetings, and all I wanted to eat was this particular salad concoction that I make at the immense Whole Foods Market salad bar in Venice, California. Lots of baby greens, loaded with a few tofu squares, plus small scoops of peas, corn, tabbouleh, hummus, shredded carrots, shredded zucchini, pickled cauliflower, and finally topped with two different items from the hot department—generally shredded BBQ chicken or Greek chicken and an Indian dish. Balsamic vinegar and a little salt and pepper finish it off. Wearing stilettos and a sun dress, I purposefully shuffled along the bar, scooping each of my items into the brown cardboard box, when a tall, dark, and handsome (I know . . .) guy stopped me.

He: *"You seem to know how to make a salad and I'm struggling here. What's a good combination?"*

I could've listed off what I included in mine, which would have been a fine answer, but I added a flirtatious slant—of course.

Me: *"I like my salads layered and interesting so that with each bite you fill your mouth with a different flavor or texture. I start with lots of greens to keep from going overboard and to create a healthy foundation. Then I choose a few select vegetables to layer in some excitement. Finally I top it with something hot to marry the flavors, add dimension, and satisfy my taste buds."*

He: *"So you like a layered and interesting salad?"*

Me: *"I do. Or else it's boring and what's the point of that? Of course, it's healthy and that's great, but healthy can also be exciting if you do it right."*

We continued to talk about the salad as if we were talking about dating. After a few minutes back and forth . . .

He: *"I'm Jack, by the way."*

Me: *"Nice to meet you, Jack. I'm Laurel,"* I said with a sideways smile.

He: *"What do you do for a living, Laurel? Something creative, I assume, based on your salad strategy."*

Me: *"I'm a writer. So yes, something creative. What about you?"*

He: *"A writer. What kind of writer? I'm an addictions therapist. And I'm trying to write a book."*

Me: *"Interesting. I write books, and one of the topics I am currently writing about is love addictions."*

He: *"Small world. I'd love to take you out sometime and talk more about your books, and maybe I can help you with the topic of love addictions."*

We exchanged business cards. Mine only has my e-mail address as my contact info, no phone number. It's strategic. When I got home I of course googled him to confirm that he wasn't a quack. That night he e-mailed me. We went out a few days later and continued to date for several months.

After that I made sure to always be on at the grocery store, and, sure enough, almost every time I go I get hit on.

* * *

Quick: you have three seconds to potentially change your life. Either you can turn that encounter with a new person into a passing, hardly noticed moment in time, or you can realize (and make him realize too) that this someone could possibly be the love of your life.

Dating is all about putting your best self forward, which starts with conversation, not small talk. Conversation isn't intended to waste time or fill space; it's meant to enrich. Even two minutes of conversation has that life-changing ability.

Whether you're the one initiating the conversation with the guy or you're being hit on at a bar, starting a conversation with an unseen stranger online or being introduced by a mutual friend at a dinner party, what you say instantly expands or shrinks (and even can shut down) your relationship potential. You have mere moments to stand out, come across as interesting, and make him want to continue to chat long enough to exchange contact information and potentially bud a relationship. So what do you say? "It's a nice day today, isn't it?" Probably not.

You want to avoid yes or no questions, but instead be immediately engaging without seeming like you're trying too hard. It's a delicate balance. How do you immediately engage? By being interesting. Don't think you're so interesting? Oh you are; everyone is. It's just picking out the interesting elements of your life—both your past and day to day—then having the confidence to bring those to life when you've got three, two, one second to make a first impression.

But being an instantly engaging and interesting conversationalist takes preparation and thought. At first you might feel like it's too much of a burden to put in the work, but soon it will become a habit and you will naturally be that person who can talk to anyone and pull people in without even trying. I'll let you in on a little secret: the majority of those people who are naturally so engaging actually fumbled at first. They practiced it. And finally, after enduring countless awkward moments, they became "naturals"—just like you will be if you put in the effort. Here's how to prepare:

Skim the news. Skim a couple of articles on websites like the *Wall Street Journal, New York Times, New York Post, Los Angeles Times, Financial Times* (which has a fantastic weekend Style section), and others that cover current events. Remember a couple of the stories and think about them for a moment so that you layer the facts with your own opinion.

Daily check-ins. Check in with yourself several times a day, thinking about what was interesting or different that you did, saw, heard, learned. What little things might be worthy of telling someone? When I say little, I mean little. Your daily check-ins will lead to elevator conversations, which we will talk about in a minute. If you don't find much that happens in your life very interesting, imagine that you have an ongoing Twitter feed reporting the shareable moments of your day. What would you post that people would actually find interesting as opposed to annoying or self indulgent? Still can't think of anything interesting? Then pay attention. Is there something interesting that you learned over the radio? A random fact that you overheard someone telling another? An out-of-the-ordinary sighting that you noticed while driving down the street? I am positive that interesting things are happening all day, all around you. You just might be too focused on something else, like looking down at your phone, to notice. Stop and smell the roses. Which translates to: pay attention to what is going on around you instead of just letting it continue to pass you by.

ELEVATOR CONVERSATIONS

What? These aren't just conversations for elevators. They are conversation starters, icebreakers, points of entry that create interest without being too long-winded. They are brief, purpose-driven stories with a beginning, middle, and end. They don't have to be fascinating, but they must be interesting.

Why? I call them elevator conversations because the elevator is the perfect place to have them. You are in a confined box for several seconds with someone you don't know. So what do you say? This is where your daily check-ins can come into play. For example:

Me: *"How's your day?"*

He: *"It's good. Busy. How's yours?"*

Me: *"Adventurous so far! I went on my daily hike this morning with my dog and we came across a huge rattlesnake on the trail. It was dead, poor guy, but my dog was excited about it! Do you ever take advantage of the hiking trails around here?"*

He: *"That's awesome that you hike every day. I've been looking for someone to hike with, since I'm new to LA. Where do you go?"*

... And the conversation has begun.

Do you think that I came across a rattlesnake this morning on the trail? I didn't, actually. But I did see it last week and I pocketed it as a great short elevator conversation that could be my point of entry.

What else did I do in those moments of conversation? I started with a setup question, assuming that his answer would be the typical "good," followed by the same question back. When I answered the question back, instead of repeating that my day was good, I said that it was "adventurous so far!" Why? Because it was an unexpected push of energy that shows that I am an exciting person who might be fun to hang out with. Then I gave my daily check-in insight and followed it up with a question to engage him back and keep the conversation flowing.

Homework: Now, I want you to have five elevator conversations a week with people who truly have real relationship (or at least date) potential.

BACK TO BASICS

What? Just say hi and introduce yourself! You don't always have to be clever. "Hello! I'm Laurel. And you are?"

Why? It's not a corny pickup line. You are offering your name first, then asking his. If he's interested, you will know because he either will or will not respond. If he's interested, it's time to start the conversation! If he isn't receptive, don't stress. He might have a girlfriend already.

ENGAGE YOUR ENVIRONMENT

What? Look around and comment on something that you see, smell, or notice, then wrap it into a story. For example, you might say, "That's an interesting ampersand art piece on the wall. It's one of my favorite symbols. Travel is a passion of mine—I actually host a travel radio show once a month in Santa Barbara, and the studio that I record in is called Ampersand. What was the last cool place you traveled to?"

Why? Having an awareness of your environment gives you bunches of conversation starters right off the bat. When you wrap it into a story, you are telling and showing a side of yourself in a relatable and engaging way that invites conversation.

THE OBVIOUS THING THAT YOU HAVE IN COMMON

What? If you just have no idea what to talk about, ask a totally open-ended question about the one thing that you both have in common.

If you're at a party, that one thing might be the host: "How do you know (enter host's name here)?"

If you're at a bar, that one thing might be the bar: "This is my first time coming here. I usually go to (X bar), but felt like trying something new. What about you?"

Why? You have no idea where this question will take you. It might take you back to stories of high school when you and the host first met. It might lead to a conversation about being a parent and knowing the host from playgroups with the kids. It might lead to a conversation about not even knowing the host, but being the fill-in date for your friend whose boyfriend broke up with her two days before Christmas—"can you believe that?!"

In the bar scenario, you are activating the power of "me too." Simply having something in common, whether it's your first time at a bar or it's your cocktail preference—a gin gimlet up—having something in common automatically makes you feel like you are connected.

What? At a bookstore? Notice the area that he is browsing: travel, fitness, art, cooking, or fiction, then strike up a conversation about it.

Why? Especially if you have knowledge about the topic, this is a great point of entry because you know that he is knowledgeable or at least interested in the topic, too. By the way, this works at wine shops, grocery stores, and really any other store too; the difference is that the topic is already focused in on what the store sells.

Start the conversation by saying

- Travel section: "A book on Istanbul?! I was there last summer and loved the spice market. Are you planning a trip there soon?"

- Fitness section: "You know, I have always wanted to try CrossFit. I was at a resort a few months ago where the author of that book was a guest teacher. I've heard guys say that CrossFit is too tough for women, but I like a challenge. What do you think? Do you think I can handle it?"

- Art section: "I have always found contemporary art intriguing, but don't know enough about it. Though I have seen *The Bean* in Chicago—which is pretty awesome. Is art a passion of yours?"

Notice that in every scenario I asked a question and also shared something about myself. Model your expectation of him by making yourself the example. I'll show you mine, then you show me yours.

Regardless of where you are, it is not only possible but important to have conversations that are somewhat substantive. Small talk might be your point of entry, but going on and on about movies, drinks, or music preferences is boring and forgettable. If you want to be memorable, dive in! I don't care if he's hot, rich, famous, or in any other way, shape, or form intimidating. He's just a guy. You are an awesome chick! Let him see how interesting you are. That doesn't mean that you should talk his ear off. But be engaging. Ask pointed questions. Listen carefully. Comment on what he says. Add your two cents. Contribute your own story. Talk about travel, exploring the world, work (if it's interesting), passions, and priorities. The point is that you want to tip-toe away from surface conversations and into topics that highlight your radiance (without looking like you're trying too hard) in order to be memorable.

SIMPLE BUT STRESSED-OVER FIRST-DATE BASICS

On the first date you set the precedent for the relationship. While the basics may seem simple, there is a reason that they are stressed over: because they matter. Let's go over a few of the basics.

WHO DOES THE FIRST DATE ASKING?

He does. Gender roles are an essential component when it comes to forming the foundation of a relationship, particularly when it comes to the first date. Men love the chase. It empowers, excites, and invigorates them. Women are alluring, pulling men in and then sitting back and accepting the hard work they put into the chase and being grateful—rewarding them for doing such a great job. However, it's okay for a woman to do the initial outreach and start the conversation. She can even hint that she'd like to go out with him or see him again. But overall, it is a man's role to do the chasing. Here's a basic breakdown:

Initial outreach: man or woman

Asking on a date: man

Paying for the date: man

Texting the day after to say thank-you: woman

Asking for a second date: man

That said, women should definitely not be passive. No one benefits from that. You are purpose driven. You can get a guy to pay attention to you, put yourself out there just enough so that he asks you out, and create an environment of trust and intrigue so that he asks you out again. In the end, he may be chasing, but you are leading the horse to water.

If you try to take hold of the reins, do the initial asking, plan the first dates, and make it "easy" for him, you are taking the thrill of the chase away, making yourself seem like you're not a prize to be worked for and

unknowingly emasculating him—all are very bad and total buzz (and rela-
tionship-potential) killers.

Don't you want him to be thinking about you all day? Don't you want
him to be strategizing how he is going to make you happy? Don't you
want him to be formulating a plan to get you to want him above all others?
Don't you want him to want to impress you? So does he. Don't take that
away from him!

WHERE NOT TO GO?

Movies, most physical activities, the theater, and coffee are all horrendous
first date activities. Here's why:

Movies: You sit next to each other in a dark room in silence. You
don't have the opportunity to talk and get to know each other,
which totally defeats the purpose of a first date. A movie isn't okay
until the third date unless you are having dinner first.

Most physical activities: Unless the activity allows for a cute outfit
or you are doing the activity first and dinner after or lunch first and
activity after, you don't want to do a physical activity. The reason is
that the first date is when you want to put your best foot forward.
In other words, you want to dress nicely, look hot, and feel even
sexier! Men feel even more manly when they are with a feminine
woman.

The theater: As fun as a first date to a musical, concert, or play
may seem, same as with a movie date—you don't have enough of
an opportunity to really get to know each other. Your focus is elsewhere, and you've set yourself up for limited conversation.

Coffee: I know, it's a go-to for so many guys because of the expense
of dates, particularly if you are a prolific dater. And although I
respect the desire to save money, coffee is overtly cheap, doesn't
usually offer the privacy to really talk about substantive things, is
not intimate in any way, and is generally too short to really get to

know anyone. Plus, it often occurs in the afternoon when lots of other things are still pending later in the day or your mind isn't clear from the meeting that you just got out of in order to make the bullshit coffee date on time. In other words, you are in an environment that totally lacks the necessities that contribute to creating intimacy, getting vulnerable and raw, forming trust, feeling connected, and leaving intrigue. It's a throwaway. Coffee dates are for casual friends, business meetings, and taking a beat to be with yourself—not first dates.

WHERE *SHOULD* YOU GO?

Dinner, drinks, a picnic, strolling around an interactive museum or even a bookstore are great first-date places where you have the opportunity to have substantive conversations, show your authentic personality and get a sense of his, share experiences and stories, connect on multiple levels, flirt, and have fun! Dating doesn't have to be expensive. Yes, spending less requires more thought, but less-expensive dates can often be the best because, when well executed, they are more creative and personalized.

If he asks you out to dinner, then says, "Where do you want to go?" instead of telling him where to take you or saying, "I don't know, you choose," give him three options of varying price and type. That way he is still being the man and making the decision, is investing in the location selection so he can also be excited about it, can get a feel for your preferences, and can do some research to see which place best accommodates his budget and the style of date that he had in mind.

HOW TO DRESS?

Dress the part. Are you dressing the part of girlfriend? One-night stand? Friend with benefits? Friend? Businesswoman? Lazy? Put some effort into your outfit. I'll say it again: a man feels more manly with a feminine woman on his arm. That doesn't mean you have to wear a pink dress. But you should dress up a bit. Wear a body-flattering outfit (like a dress or cute blouse with butt-enhancing jeans), do your hair, put some makeup on, wear high heels. I'm not being sexist. I'm saying to put some effort into your look in order to present your best self. Be a sexy woman!

Men are visual creatures. Your first impression—which includes appearances, is essential. Every time you go out, wear one thing that is eye catching and makes you stand out. It can be your signature color (pink or red or electric blue to pull out your eyes), a cool hat, burgundy stilettos, etc. Make a statement, but don't be shocking. Wear something that will get you noticed but that you are also comfortable in. If it helps, on a day when you are at home with nothing to do and you're feeling sassy and sexy, go into your closet and design five to ten go-to outfits that you know look good on you. Write them down or take a photo so that you don't have to stress about it later. Take note when you wear something different and people compliment you on it. Is it men or women who notice and compliment? Look around and see what types of outfits catch your eye. What is it about the outfit that draws your attention? Try to emulate it within your own style.

WHAT TO EAT AND DRINK?

Drinks date: The problem with drinks dates is that you don't know whether you should eat first. What if drinks turns into dinner and you already ate?! What if you don't know if it will turn into dinner, so you don't eat . . . and then it's just drinks and you get drunk? Have a base food. Something substantive but low enough in calories that you can eat dinner also and not feel full or that can help create a base in case there is no dinner. A few ideas? A Balance Bar, banana, or yam. Once you're on the date, it's fine to have a couple of drinks. Just know your tolerance level and by all means *don't* pass it! You do *not* want to be that drunk girl on a date. Stay in control, but drop your guard enough to be real and emotionally available.

Dinner date: Don't order like a girl. Eat! Guys are generally turned off by prissy women who are über-picky eaters, eat only salads, or order food just to pick at it without actually eating anything. Order what you would normally order when out to dinner, being cognizant of the price of the items. Before you place your order, ask him what he's thinking about so you can gauge whether he is getting an entrée and a starter or just an entrée. If he is getting a starter, then you should select one too, the reason being that it's awkward for you to sit and watch him as he eats his starter alone while you wait for him to finish before your entrées are sent out.

WHO PAYS?

He does. Always. Friends go Dutch. Business associates go Dutch. Dates don't. What do you want? A friend? A business partner? A job? Or a boyfriend that might lead to a husband? Do not pay. Do not offer to pay. Do not do the fake reach for your wallet. Guys pay on the first date. Period. End of story. I don't care if you are wealthier, uglier, fatter, less popular, more pathetic, or luckier (to be out with him than he is with you). You are the woman. Your presence and radiance is payment enough on that first date. In fact, it's payment enough on the first several dates (if not all dates).

That being said, you can pay in other ways on other dates—like cooking dinner and buying the ingredients—which is also a serious turn-on, as it shows that you are a nurturer. Even if you suck at cooking, it truly is the thought that counts. Have a special something arranged, like schedule a couples massage or a cocktail-making class, or arrange an activity like a picnic with wine and an amazing cheese assortment that you pick up from a specialty grocery store. You can be responsible for atypical dates. But pulling out a credit card or cash from your wallet at the dinner table is a masculine act, and it is not for a feminine woman to do. Paying = providing (masculine). Cooking or gifting = nurturing (feminine).

Now, I'm not saying to go on that date and be a bitch, act entitled, or be dismissive. No. Be sweet, interesting (contribute to the conversation), interested (in what he has to say), effervescent, sassy, whatever you are—be you. But be a confident you. Be your best you.

You're an independent traditionalist, but he's still paying. Now, to clarify, just because he is paying, doesn't mean that you are not a strong, self-sufficient, independent woman. This isn't about independence. It isn't about your ability to buy your own dinner and pay your own way. This is about gender roles and chivalry. Yes, you are an independent traditionalist. Men and women may be equals, but we are not the same; we have our own roles and contribute in our own ways.

Another clarification: just because he is paying doesn't mean that you owe him *anything* after.

Let him feel like he scored! By letting him pay, you are allowing him to feel a huge amount of pride. As odd as it might sound, when a guy walks into a restaurant with a woman on his arm he feels lucky to be with, he feels like he owns the place! The food that you order: he feels like he prepared it for you. And that's a great thing. You want him to take pride in you. So act like he should. If you offer to pay, you are essentially saying, "I don't deserve for you to pay." You are automatically demoting yourself. Your guy should feel just slightly luckier to be with you. Why? Because guys are the ones who tend to have wandering eyes (while women have wandering minds). A guy wants to feel like he won the prize, like he's the big man on campus, with the most desired chick on his arm. Let him feel like he scored! Let him feel that way and even if you are uglier, fatter, less popular, he scored. He scored you. You know it, so he will believe it. He is paying on that first date.

Now, in the same breath, don't act like a gold digger. Be cognizant of price. Don't select a date spot that is crazy expensive. Don't order the priciest item on the menu. Don't take advantage of the situation. As soon as he plops down the money, you will say in a very sweet way, as you look him in the eyes and warmly smile—"thank you."

WHAT NEXT?

Sending a post-date thank-you text is essential if you liked the guy and would like to see him again. Yes—*you* send that first text. Here's why: the guy planned and paid for dinner. Men, like dogs, do things on the reward system. If he does something you like, you reward him by letting him know he did a great job. Think about how men are at work. If they put in a little extra effort, they are rewarded by a compliment from the boss, a "great job" handshake, and eventually maybe a raise or a promotion. If his extra work goes unnoticed, the guy isn't going to continue to make the effort. Why would he? He *wants* to please you. Reward him by telling him that you had a great time and you look forward to seeing him again. Sending a text to say thank-you isn't being too forward. In fact, it's a very feminine thing to do—to show gratitude. You are expressing your appreciation. Don't stress about it. Just do it.

You may think online dating is fun and games. And although it certainly can be fun, it's not a game if you want to find love online; it's a strategy. What's the difference? Games are about manipulation. Strategy is about smarts.

That said, online dating can be intimidating, feel like a waste of your time, or seem like a cesspool filled with gross, low-quality men. Let me tell you that you're not alone if

- you feel like you're throwing spaghetti at the walls, hoping something will stick;
- you feel like there are no good, high-quality prospects who are your type;
- you wonder why you're getting few to zero responses;
- you can't figure out what you're doing wrong;
- you've had a bad experience with it and are therefore repelled by it; or
- you believe that the best way to meet your Mr. Right is "naturally," where you will have a better gauge of your chemistry before committing to a date, and you might be dismissive of it.

Get over it.

Be prepared to be a little overwhelmed—at first. I am about to give you a lot of information. Some of the tips are simple tweaks, others are a shift in thought processes, or it might feel like a total overhaul. But I promise you, they are all practical, easy-to-follow, actionable, tested, and proven-to-work insights that you will quickly get the hang of and put into use to dramatically change your confidence and success dating online.

Because the fact is that online dating can be one of the most efficient ways to find your Mr. Right (or even Mr. Right Now). It can also be a total time-, energy-, and money-sapping experience that feels more like a full-time job than a fun way to get out there and meet your match.

The purpose of online dating is to show and tell who you are and what a life with you would look like. Think about how you are presenting yourself. The person you want to present should be the best version of yourself. Maybe your day to day right now as an overworked single woman is pretty boring. But is that what you always want your life to be like? If you were in a relationship, would you still have all of the same old boring routines? Before you can put forward an honest, but best, version of yourself, I need you to first be honest *with* yourself. This is why we put in all the self-analyzing work at the beginning of this book—so that you could figure out who you truly are at your core, what you stand for as a person, what you actually enjoy doing, what your dating purpose is, and what you really NEED as opposed to what you WANT.

Now let's get you online.

SETTING UP YOUR PROFILE

Don't look at this as your opportunity to create the ultimate advertisement to sell yourself. Sure, that's an element of your online profile, but, more than that, it's an invitation to certain guys—the right guys—and a repellant to the wrong guys. One of the most important but often ignored elements of online dating is elimination. The way you write your profile as well as the way that you prequalify your potential dates are great opportunities to narrow the playing field. That's right, you *want* to narrow it. Because the goal of online dating isn't to attract everyone; it's to attract the right one. Here are a few dos and don'ts:

> **DO** be totally honest about who you are and what you are looking for. Why? Because you want to cut out the people who will, in the end, be a waste of your time because they aren't right for you and never were from the very beginning. For example, if you say that you are a lover of "the finer things in life" and you "feel sexiest in a pair of Christian Dior stilettos but can also rock a comfy James Perse white T-shirt and go out for a slice of pizza" . . . guys who appreciate—and likely guys who can afford—seven-hundred-dollar shoes and have heard of James Perse will find that a turn-on. Men who, on the contrary, are turned off by a woman who likes

expensive stuff will probably not contact you. And that's a good thing. Because if you're being honest with yourself, you want the guy who understands and maybe even can provide for your lifestyle preferences. Some guys are looking for their little princess. If you are outdoorsy, love to go camping, can't stand high heels, and consider yourself to be a bit of a tomboy, great! Say that! Don't be brash or rude. Be you. If you have a sarcastic side, slip that in too! If you're witty, if you pride yourself on your wisdom, if your spirituality is a major component of who you are, or if you are a total movie geek—say it! You are not here to please everyone. You are trying to please yourself first by weeding out the guys who might take issue with elements of who you are and what expectations you have.

DO start with something that sets you apart. A great way to do that is by setting up a challenge at the beginning. Like what? Start with a quote. Then at the top of your profile, challenge the viewer to tell you who said it. If he instantly knows the answer—well, you've already got one thing in common! He just might google it if he's up for the challenge, even if he isn't particularly interested.

For example: "And in the end ... The love you take ... is equal to the love ... you make." Followed up with: "If you can identify the author of my headline, you get extra points. If you live those words every day, you get double extra points, and I want to hear from you immediately."

DO reveal your core values. Reveal something about yourself that comes from your core values, your essence, who you really are. Share something fun or funny about yourself. The last thing you want to write is a bland, canned, throwaway profile that says nothing. The purpose is to start pulling back the layers of your onion, exposing a side of you that makes the reader feel like he has seen something that might not come across in your photos or maybe something that makes him feel like he gets you, and definitely something that makes him intrigued by you. By opening up just a little, you are showing him that you are a real person who is layered and interesting and someone he really wants to get to know better.

You are also starting to create that essential environment of trust that makes him feel safe enough to start revealing himself to you too.

DON'T state what you're *not* looking for. That should be apparent in what you *are* looking for.

DON'T say that you are looking to get married (like yesterday), knocked up tomorrow, and already have the minivan on hold for the soccer team of kids that you're looking to pop out.

DON'T be rude, offensive, political, preachy, slutty, or crude.

DON'T cuss.

DON'T make spelling errors.

NAME

This is generally the first thing that a potential suitor sees. It should say something about who you are and what you stand for. It shouldn't be "lovergirl154" (it's cheesy and slutty), or "12345" (how boring and unmemorable), or "thisislame" (*that* is lame), or "cantthinkofaname" (that's because you aren't putting any effort into it), or "pickme" (desperate), or "LaurelHouse" (you don't want to reveal who you are). Never, never, never use your real name! Your name doesn't have to be deep. But it should have some type of meaning, because chances are you will be asked about it.

To come up with a name, ask yourself this question: "Who am I?" If you define yourself by your career and your location—use those. For example:

- A writer who is proud of her Los Angeles roots: "LAwriterGirl"
- A chef who is originally from Paris: "FrenchyFoodie"
- If you love both fitness and high fashion, maybe "SneaksToStilettos"
- If you are super into literature, choose a short quote from your favorite author

- If you have both dogs and cats and take the "must love dogs and cats" approach, try "purrwoof"

Remember, once you decide on a name, if you go off the site for a bit because you found your match, then you come back on, you generally can't change your name. So put some thought into making it timeless.

TAGLINE

Similar to your name, put some effort into it. Since you are allowed spaces in between the words, you can actually say something of a bit more substance. Quotes are great here. Your goal for online dating works too (as long as it's not "I want kids now!"). This is also your opportunity to divulge a bit about who you are and what you stand for. It can also explain your name—as the subtitle of a book might do. A tagline that stimulates conversation, that makes him think, or that asks a thought-provoking question is ideal, as it can be used as an opener in initial outreach and also shows that he's actually read your profile.

For example:

- Interesting and interested
- Let's get off, and stay off, online dating
- Real
- Wickedly smart is so sexy
- Click HERE to add to cart
- Happy, sweet, and always an adventure
- Yoga, cupcakes, relaxing, and going, going . . . it's a balance
- Happy as me, happier as we

PHOTOS

DO post at least five. Your photos should show and tell who you are.

DO post a couple of headshot-type photos that clearly show your face and features.

DO post at least one full-body shot (not in a swimsuit).

DO post photos of you smiling and having fun!

DO post photos of you doing activities.

DO post photos of you both dressed up and dressed down.

DON'T post more than one photo of you with an alcoholic drink in your hand.

DON'T post selfies of yourself in the mirror.

DON'T post photos of you with other guys (guys naturally get jealous).

DON'T post photos with other girls (guys naturally compare).

This is just the tip of the iceberg when it comes to online dating photos. I want to share them all with you but have only so much space in this book. You can find more on my website: ScrewingTheRules.com.

"ABOUT ME" AND "WHAT I'M LOOKING FOR"

The two are often bundled together on online dating sites. That is great, actually, because it allows you to weave them together in your description.

DON'T make it too long. It shouldn't be more than five paragraphs or one page single-spaced.

DON'T make it too short. It should be more than one paragraph.

DO tell and show. Explain who you are, then give an example of what you mean.

DO be honest.

DO proofread and spell-check.

DO be thoughtful and thought out.

As I expressed at the beginning of this section, this is your opportunity to lure in the right person and ward off the wrong person.

ANALYZING HIS PHOTOS
(AND LOOKING BEYOND THE FACE)

When checking out prospective online dates, the first stop is generally the photos. You flip through each picture, looking at his features, checking out his activities, trying to get a read on whether he looks like a nice guy, a happy guy, a fun guy, a player, or a smart guy. We all have our things in mind that we want to see. It's time to reprogram our photo analysis.

First of all, the photos shouldn't even be factored into your initial analysis. His actual profile—who he is, what he does, what his lifestyle is like, what his beliefs and needs are . . . Those are much more substantive and important. After that come the photos. And still, while flipping through his images, don't look at him first. Look past him.

What do the photos say about who he is? Where is he? What kind of environments is he in? Is he sporty, into travel, an adventurer, sophisticated, a homebody? Does he have pets? What kind of clothes is he wearing? What about his watch and shoes? Is there a car or a house in the background? What does his body language say? What is he doing? What's he holding? Is he always drinking, smoking, partying? Who is he with? Do his photos look like professional head shots? Are they head shots that look like he is an actor or model, or are they head shots that professionals like attorneys and brokers sometimes take to put up on the firm's website? Does he have children or is he photographed with other people's children? What about parents, siblings, and extended family—are they in the photos?

All of those elements add up, in part, to who he is. Sometimes they even clue you in to components of him that he didn't mean to reveal. They are also great conversation starters. Looking past the man, almost removing him from the photo, can be one of your strongest ways to collect data on him and give you a sneak peek into what the life of this man is really like.

ESSENTIAL PREQUALIFYING STRATEGY TO NEVER HAVE A BAD FIRST ONLINE DATE AGAIN

One of the best things about online dating is the opportunity to extensively prequalify the guy before going out with him. Of course, you can also prequalify if you meet the old-fashioned way (in person), but online gives you the extra edge because you first see his profile basics, you can ask many more strategic questions than you might in person, and you can even do additional research (which I recommend for both safety and more thorough prequalifying)—all of this before you have the first e-mail exchange or phone call. Traditional prequalifying starts with meeting him in person. Then you might e-mail, but more likely you'll have a phone call, followed by setting up a date, and finally texting. Like peeling back an onion, each form of communication lends itself to a different type of information extraction—as we talked about in the communication section.

ONLINE PREQUALIFYING STEP #1: PROFILE MAPPING

If you want to stop wasting a ton of time chatting with a ridiculous number of men who, let's be honest, you wouldn't give even a second glance to if you met them the old-fashioned way, then, before filling in your profile, uploading your photos, and putting yourself on the public market, you've got to "map" his profile. In other words, you are creating a standard (which I will explain in a minute) in which your eye moves across his profile—like eye mapping. Once you create the standard, you will map every guy's profile the same way, following your list of priorities so that each guy is being judged by the same criteria.

Setting a standard: What are your priorities—looks, career, humor, intellect, interests, money, edge, religion, geographic location, etc.? Hopefully in the sections "Screw Tall, Dark, and Handsome" and "Stop Looking for What You Want and Get What You Need," you had the opportunity to hone in on what type of guy is the best fit for you.

Devising a plan: Your standards will help dictate what specifically you are looking for in their profiles. Since you *are* sticking with your standards and mapping each man in the same way, if your main criteria aren't fulfilled . . . delete. For example, if you have a certain standard of living that you are looking for (i.e., money), and he checked the box that says that he doesn't make much, X him out immediately. Why be so shallow? It's not shallow; you're simply being honest with yourself. Otherwise, you might know you want a rich guy, but you go on several dates with the poor guy. After a month you simply aren't getting what you want, so you have to break it off. But you knew that already, even before you accepted the date. Same goes for career, the desire to have kids, smoking, religion, and proximity. Why set your relationship up for disappointment by dating someone who you know right off the bat can't provide what you need? Because you are judging each profile based on the same standard—determined by your priorities—it is easier to stay on-purpose. Once you get the hang of profile mapping, you will be able to quickly ease your eyes over each guy's profile, determining whether he's a pass or whether you are going to promote him to the next level: communication.

PREQUALIFYING STEP #2: COMMUNICATION

It's totally acceptable for you to do the first outreach. If you see a guy you're interested in, instead of sitting there wishing and hoping and praying and waiting and obsessing and getting depressed and derailing yourself, send him a message! But don't just send some lame "Hi, I saw your profile and I would love to get to know you" message. Could that be any more generic, thoughtless, and cardboard? That's an excellent way to be overlooked and ignored. Instead, say something that will make you stand out and shows that you put some thought into it. But you don't want to appear like you sat and slaved over your message for hours as you assault him with way too much information that he has no interest in reading. Annoyed at the multiple paragraphs that he knows will take way too much time to read, he'll simply hit delete. Here's how you can start the conversation:

Where are you from? "Hello! Where are you from originally? I'm one of the few Angelenos actually born and bred in Los Angeles. What about you? What brought you to LA?" Statistically, "Where are you from originally?" has a 75 percent better chance of getting a reply than an average message—that's according to the online dating website AYI.com. Why? Because it's a question that isn't cheesy, doesn't seem canned, and every single person can relate to with a substantive answer. People love to talk about themselves, but in the very initial stages of communication we don't want to feel like we are revealing too much. Where we are from is safe but still informative, and it taps into the simple desire to share who we truly are.

What inspired you? You don't have to stick with "Where are you from?" to elicit an initial response. Ask other nonthreatening yet personalized and revealing questions like "So I see that you're a (insert his career here). What inspired you to go into that career?" The key word here is "inspired." People love to be, feel, and talk about being inspired. It makes us feel like we have greater purpose, even if we truly did go into law to make a lot of money.

Here are five key elements to a good icebreaking question

Always ask a question. If you just make a statement, you are making it harder for him to respond. Engage him. *Always* make sure to ask a question in your message, regardless of whether it's the first or fifth communication. Wonder why some of your past communication has fallen off? You may have neglected to ask a question that invites a response and keeps the conversation going.

Personalize the question. Not sure what to say? You've got plenty of starting topics to choose from in his profile. For example, "I see that you like to cook. What was the last delicious meal that you made?" or "You seem to be an avid reader. What book are you reading now, and what inspired you to pick it up?" If you refer to something in his profile—like his career, his favorite destination, a book he read, a physical activity he enjoys—it shows that you took the time to read it, as opposed to just looking at the photos.

Reveal something brief about yourself. This isn't just an interview. You are opening the lines of communication and connection, as well as setting the standard of expectation. If you want him to reveal, you have to reveal first.

Never just say, "You're hot. Want to meet up?" Yes, it's a question that is based on the photos in his profile and it's personalized, but it's creepy and it totally ignores the prequalifying questions that are an absolute must before you go on that first date. Even saying, "I'm intrigued" isn't okay . . . because you aren't engaging him. You are saying nothing.

Keep the initial outreach short and tight. Don't be too verbose in an attempt to sell yourself. Keeping it tight means making the words count and staying purpose driven. Don't wander or speak in circles. Or worse—don't say nothing at all. Within your brevity, you need to make sure that you stand out, particularly if you're reaching out to good-looking guys who are likely inundated with messages.

For example, "When you cook, do you cook by the taste or follow a recipe? I always try to follow recipes, but for some reason my mother's voice stirs in the back of my head saying, 'I think its missing something.' Then I am off to determine the missing element, and the recipe is tossed to the side. I wonder what that says about me. . . . "

Why does it work? It's short, addresses an interest mentioned in his profile, asks a question, shows a mutual interest, and opens up the conversation to food—which can lead to talking about going on a date. Lastly, it gets him wondering what type of person you are.

Another example: "I love that photo of you and your dog on the hike. But I definitely see snow around you guys, and you mentioned that you live in Santa Monica. Did you and your pup go on a road trip together? I took my dog Daisy on a cross-country trip once. Well, we were moving from New York. She was a surprisingly great travel companion. It was the first time I took a trip alone (without people), and it was incredibly inspiring. Have you ever traveled alone?"

Why does it work? You asked a question about road trips, brought attention to your shared pup companion, told a brief story that creates several conversation starters, and then asked another question.

PREQUALIFYING QUESTIONS TO VET HIM BEFORE GIVING ANY PERSONAL INFO

"What do you do and why?"

Purpose: It's time to think about dating strategically. "What do you do?" reveals status, true, but you're not going to be dating his status; you're going to be dating his career along with him. Translation: his personality, hours, vacations, date nights, the way you're treated, the way he expects to be treated, his bedroom demeanor, how you dress (from camo miniskirts and crossbone tees to couture three-quarter-sleeve jackets and tweed, the requisite clothing for dating a rock star versus an executive. I know, it's extreme, but I actually experienced them back to back), overall your daily and long-term life will all be dictated by his career. His career type is a type generalization that reveals much more than his sign, clothing style, car, height, and looks do. What does your guy spend the majority of his time attending to? His career. If his career doesn't match your personality, if the lifestyle it requires doesn't align with what you have determined appropriate for you, if you simply can't stand what your guy does for a living, maybe he's not the one. After all, in addition to taking up his time and requiring his attention, he choose that career, decided that he wanted to live that lifestyle, put in those hours, and will spend the rest of his days plugging away doing that. Says something about someone, doesn't it?

"Tell me five random things about you that you find most interesting."

Purpose: Unless he takes it as a joke, he will likely think about this one for a second and tell you some pretty interesting and introspective things—revealing things. He may share his education, honors, lifestyle, upbringing, talents, idiosyncrasies, taste, social status, or quirks. It may also reveal things that are on your must-have or won't-stand list that will immediately turn you on or off. The answers to this question may make you decide to stop responding to him and move on—*or* make you even more intrigued.

"What does your average day/week/month look like?"

Purpose: The success of this question depends on the openness of the guy. He very well can rush and brush this one off. But if he takes it seriously, it can reveal what his work/life balance is like, whether he has pets, whether he travels, how often he hangs out with friends, whether he has any hobbies, how close he is to his family, whether he has a roommate or lives alone, and what his living situation is (house, apartment, backyard, etc.). In other words, it reveals things that are important to him and take priority in his daily life.

"Why?"

Purpose: I'm not asking you a question. Nor am I setting up an answer. That's the answer: "Why?" What's great about "Why?" is that it's a question you can tack onto almost any other mundane question and suddenly transform it into something substantive and revealing. It allows you to better understand his perspective and point of view. Why does he think that way? Why does he feel that way? Why does he have an interest in that topic? It's not just about communication, it's about learning about him, and therefore learning whether he's right for you. Asking why allows for the opportunity to open up, delve deeper into subjects that he might normally not talk about, and maybe even tap into a raw and vulnerable side that he isn't accustomed to exploring. By asking why (in a nonthreatening and unpatronizing way, of course), you are expressing true interest. Plus, you will be able to understand the root of decisions and passions and the impetus for his interests.

Here are a few examples in which "Why?" completely transforms a surface topic into something that's revealing:

- "Why did you decide to be a doctor?"
- "Why do you love romance movies?"
- "Why do you love photography as a hobby?"
- "Why did you decide to move from New York to Los Angeles?"
- "Why does your family eat tamales on Christmas instead of a traditional turkey or ham?"

"What do you like to do for your partner to make her feel loved?
What makes you feel loved?"

Purpose: This one may seem like an odd question, but everyone has his or her own way of showing affection—for some it's being touchy-feely or simply spending time together, for others it's gifts, and for others it's offering advice and help in business. It's also important to understand what he thinks it is that makes him feel loved so that you can have an understanding of what is expected of you. For example, spending time together, the little things, a home-cooked dinner, conversation, a back rub, etc. The answer can also simply allow you insight into the mind of a man.

OTHER GOOD QUESTIONS

Here are some more good ones that might not say a lot about the guy as a person or address any components on your priorities list. But they will be fun to learn and will reveal a bit about his interests and sensibility.

- "What's your favorite flavor of ice cream and why?"
- "What's your favorite movie/book and why?"
- "What's your favorite time of year and why?"
- "What's the best gift you ever received growing up and why?"
- "What's your favorite dorky moment and why?"
- "What three apps on your phone do you use the most and why?"

Tip. Notice that it's the "and why" part of the question that is essential, or else you will likely get an answer like "French silk ice cream"—which must have a story to it because it's kind of an obscure favorite, but you didn't ask why. Or worse, the answer could simply be "vanilla"—something so plain and so susceptible to judgment that you might even be inclined to shut him out right then! But what if the "why" is because he's "obsessed with toppings and vanilla is the perfect blank slate . . . "? That's a pretty interesting and compelling reason to let him stick around.

QUESTIONS THAT REALLY ASK NOTHING

And then there are those questions that reveal pretty much nothing yet are all too common. Sure, they reveal an answer, but what does that answer really say about him? Remember: the goal of your questions is to extract enough information to determine whether you are interested in going out with him and minimizing the chance that your date will be a total waste.

- "What kinds of music do you like?" This one is a dud because really, who cares what kind of music you like? Unless he's a musician it's nonsubstantive and expresses nothing.

- "Where do you like to vacation?" Again, who cares? You both like beach vacations—yay! Yeah right. Unless you tack on the "why?" question, what type of vacations you prefer reveals nothing of depth and sounds more like you're ready for a fun, not for a real, relationship.

- "What are you looking for in a relationship partner?" This is way too broad and hard to put into specific words. It's like asking, "What's up?" Unlike the specific question of "What makes you feel loved?" which can reveal whether you feel most loved when you are given little presents, given a lot of time, or hearing sweet nothings, "What are you looking for?" is too grand of a question and often will elicit a list of wants as opposed to needs, which again are generally surface and not substantive.

LOVE IS A SKYSCRAPER—
GO DOWN BEFORE YOU GO UP

When it comes to getting a guy to fall in love with you—deep, hard, and fast—*this* is the secret miracle strategy: go down before you go up.

Relationships that end quickly are often built on superficial grounds. You think, "He's so hot," "I love his car," "Look at his body," "He's hysterical," "He's so much fun," ... And you fall in love with that, not him. If you want to build a love that lasts, think about a skyscraper.

Before skyscrapers reach their impressive mile heights, the foundation is formed several stories beneath the ground. If, instead, the builders decided to screw putting in the work and constructed from the ground up, although it might appear stunning at first, that building is destined to come tumbling down. Same goes for relationships. Go down before you go up. Sure, his abs are washboard delicious, but that's not reason enough to hook up. What else is there to him? Who is he really? Can you have a conversation of substance? Try to understand who he is as a human being. What are his core values, and do they align with yours?

So how do you get him to expose his truths when he doesn't even know you?

THE U FALL IN LOVE STRATEGY

This three-step strategy is structured to open up both you and him, allowing you to see each other as your best, most authentic selves—which sets the stage to feel and fall in love.

First, compliment his façade. You see each other, in your presentation form, as pretty spectacular, or you wouldn't have wanted to go out in the first place. That's the top of the "U."

Then, get raw. Yes, even on the first date. One of the most efficient and effective ways to dip down deep into that U and bring a guy's walls down is to bring yours down first. Like Miley Cyrus's song "Wrecking Ball" says, "I came in like a wrecking ball / . . . All I wanted was to break your walls / . . . I just wanted you to let me in / And instead of using force / I guess I should have let you in." Reveal a story about yourself, and he will respond with a story in kind, following you down into his depths. Be open and real so that you can get to know each other in that stripped-down state. Now you've got him vulnerable and exposed.

Finally, make him feel like a god. Next, you build him up and make him feel amazing—because knowing what you now know about him and his authentic self, you truly feel that he *is* amazing. And he will affix to you like a barnacle to a boat.

SCREW CHEMISTRY. IS THERE A CONNECTION?

What's the purpose of a first date? To decide whether this guy has any possibility of being appropriate for you, and you for him. It's also your first opportunity to gauge whether there's any pull between you two, whether there's chemistry, attraction, a connection. Although chemistry and attraction may be instant and they may be the immediate hit of fireworks that draws you in, their depths are shallow and even dangerous. Sure, attraction and chemistry are important. But they can be blinding. If you fall for someone based on that shallow rush, you might not see (or you might ignore) the deeper, more substantive characteristics and core values that truly do create that deep bond—the bond that builds and endures, as opposed to one of those fun and fast fireworks that thrill you for a moment, and might even feel like the real thing at first, and then just as quickly fade away.

Set the standard. You are setting the standard and establishing the expectation. Oftentimes women allow the guy to set the tone. We follow how he communicates with us. And that's the exact wrong way to get a guy to open up and be revealing with you.

Create an environment of trust and a safe space for honesty. You've got to show him who you are first, then he will follow your lead and show you what he has hiding beneath his tough-guy façade. Knowing each other on a deep and real level reveals that "secret side" that few people get to see.

Establish understanding and respect. Once you are both wide open, you will have more respect for each other. You will see each other's triumphs as even more remarkable because you have an understanding of what you have each overcome to obtain them. You are pulling down your walls and showing the inner workings, the painstaking experiences, and the reality of who you are and what you went through to get to this amazing other side. And then comes the final upswing of the U Fall in Love Strategy—you build each other back up with sincere compliments that make you both feel amazing, trusted, and respected.

You are memorable and enticing. You could be the most beautiful, successful, smartest, funniest, sweetest woman with a drool-worthy body and a wit that never lacks in comebacks. But you're not enticing. You're not alluring. You're not seductive. You're not sexy. Once you show that other side of you, that raw side, that passionate side, that vulnerable side, then you start to be sexy, then you start to show depth, then you start to make him interested in what's hiding deep inside you, then you make him want to know and explore more . . . and now you're memorable and enticing.

WHAT DO YOU REVEAL?

Digging deeper into the basic U Fall in Love Strategy is the U Reveal Strategy. This is where you are exposing your vulnerability and pulling your walls down without bringing the conversation down right along with them. You want to expose an experience from your past that may have been embarrassing, painful, or something you regret or you're not proud of, but that's not to say that you should be a bummer and dwell on your old issues. Talk about what happened, expressing true emotion around it, then bring the conversation back up by explaining what you learned and how you are better or more evolved because of it. Here's what you reveal:

Your core values. But you aren't just listing your values. Instead, you are using your framed stories, which we already went over, to both show and tell your core values while simultaneously creating interesting conversation.

Pain points and vulnerabilities. When revealing things that you aren't so proud of, that you may regret, and that shaped who you are, you are letting him see the real you, not the façade of a person you create for protective purposes.

Your red flags and excess baggage. But hide your dirty laundry. There is a difference. Dirty laundry is current. Red flags and emotional baggage have been worked through and healed from. Revealing your red flags and baggage isn't just for the sake of getting it off your chest; it also can elicit even more respect from him as he comes to more deeply understand your past hardships and all that you have overcome to arrive here. With understanding comes connection. Because you're real. You are revealing your humanity and making yourself more relatable. I know, it's scary to expose those not-so-pleasant sides of yourself, but if you want him to fall in love with you, you have to tap his heart first. And you do that by making him feel. For example, if you say something like "I'm divorced. Twice, actually. I was young and not ready—both times. Twenty-one the first time, and it only lasted for six months. I was trying to have what my parents have—they were married at twenty-one and are still happily together. My second husband, we really didn't take the time to get to know each other. . . . " Do you think that's appropriate? The answer is *Yes! Absolutely!* Why? Because being divorced twice could be a red flag for someone. Don't you want to know that now, before you invest in the relationship, before you open your heart and dedicate your days? You want to be raw and honest and revealing, not just for the sake of dumping your baggage on the table but instead to say "And I have learned so much about love and what I am looking for." You fess up to having made mistakes, which shows vulnerability, but then you show the silver lining—the lessons you learned and how you are better because of it—that shows strength! That *says* something. That's real. And if he still says, " You know, the fact that you were married twice, that's a red flag for me and I can't date you," that's okay. If elements of who you are, what you have done, and where you have been are deal-breaking red flags for him, you've spared yourself time and heartbreak. There are (no joke!) plenty of fish in the sea, and you will find someone else who finds it attractive that you were open to taking a chance, to throwing caution to the wind, to jumping into love feet first . . . even if it unfortunately bit you on the butt.

Your passions. When expressing your passions, your true personality bubbles up! Your face brightens, your voice elevates, and yet another secret side is revealed. Just be careful not to go on and on about how much you are obsessed with cats, Hello Kitty, the color pink, or even *Star Wars*. If he doesn't share your enthusiasm, you might lose him after the initial interest to know more.

Your childhood. It's great to reveal a story or two from your childhood that he might be able to relate to as well. If it's funny, awkward, and embarrassing—even better! Those childhood experiences often have an effect on the person you grow up to become, so expressing those stories might give him a deeper understanding of and sensitivity to your unique traits and idiosyncrasies.

Your family. Do you have siblings? Are you close with your parents? Did your dad raise you to love camping—an annual tradition that you did with his buddies and their boys, infusing you with enthusiasm for the outdoors and campfire songs (the snake in the outhouse you could have lived without though)? Did you and your mom grow close because she forced you to hike with her every Sunday for three hours, giving you no out to be an avoidant teen until finally you "broke" and started spilling your emotional guts to her in the safety of that space? Talk about it!

If you want to find that deep, guttural love, the love that lasts, that hooks your heart and implants itself in your soul, you've got to screw the façade, the protective layer, the walls, the hiding of the feelings, and the front. You have to be raw.

BUT YOU COULD GET HURT...

When you're being vulnerable and raw and honest, you are also opening yourself up to possibly get hurt. You are exposed. You are letting him see your honest self, a side of you that not everyone is allowed access to. And he might not like it. He might view your experiences as unwanted baggage and your fears as weakness. But the benefit outweighs the possible bummer of rejection. Because, well, (1) you don't want that shallow guy anyway and it's better to find that out now! and (2) don't you want those butterflies and that true, deep, guttural love? Take the restraints off your heart and allow yourself to feel.

TALK ABOUT YOUR EX

Talk about your ex on the first date. Yes, that chunk of your life is no longer an off-limits topic of conversation. Conversations about exes are actually incredibly revealing while simultaneously setting a standard of expectation. What can ex-talk expose about you?

- The types of men you have dated and the benefits that you enjoyed because of them, which establishes a set of experience-based expectations

- Your attitude toward the opposite sex (through the way in which you talk about your ex)

- Your current state of being and readiness to be in a new, healthy relationship

- How introspective you are and your ability to look at your mistakes and missteps, and extract the lessons

- Your red flags

- How interesting you are

Plus, you show what a great catch you are. Because—let's be honest—if you dated a rock star, billionaire, head of a major company, and model, and then you're dating this guy, you are pretty much elevating his status in his mind. You can get all of them, but you are choosing him!? Instant ego booster. Simultaneously, you are motivating him to step it up a notch—which can be a good thing.

And once you bring up your ex, encourage him to chime in about his. That way, all that you revealed and the insight he potentially gained will be reciprocated.

But before going on and on about how amazing your ex was in bed and how you're pretty sure he was the love of your life—or what a shitty guy he was and how you're all but ruined because of him, read these dos and don'ts.

DO talk about the most interesting men you have dated.

Why? This lets him know you're wanted by extraordinary men and you're choosing to spend your time with him. But don't talk about this fascinating ex of yours in a way that makes it sound like you're still pining for him. Give a balanced description, including just a couple of top-level points that describe what made him so awesome and a couple of top-level points that show why you did not work as a couple and what you learned about yourself because of that relationship or experience.

DO mention a few of the amazing things that being with that ex afforded you, be it gifts, trips, introductions, associations, or experiences.

Why? You have seen and done and received and experienced on an elevated level. What you are doing is setting a standard and expectation. Sure, this new guy might not be a rock star or a millionaire or a member of Mensa, but there is a certain level of life that you have for a time been accustomed to. Letting him know this will get him thinking about what he can do to also impress and woo you. But don't go on and on. Only briefly mention a couple of things without going into details. Brush strokes are key. You're not trying to make him too jealous here—"too" being the operative word. You also don't want to make him feel like shit, like he's not good enough, or like you're a bitch. It's a balancing act. Tread lightly.

DO express regrets, share pain points and personal disappointments, and let him know that you are a real person who makes mistakes. But the key here is then expressing that you learned from those regrets, pain, and disappointments.

Why? This is an opportunity to open your heart, let him in, and reveal a real side of you that not many people get to see, which makes him feel special and trusted. When you confide in each other in this way, you are creating an environment for the formation of trust and true connection on a deep level.

DO get him to express a story or two about an ex too.

Why? First, lots of people have a thing about ex-talk. He may be one of them. However, if he reveals something about an ex too, he has now shared in a way that he didn't expect could be so healing and enlightening. If he doesn't get on the same ex-talk page, you might be annoyed that you "overshared," but not if he takes part too.

Second, this isn't just about tit for tat. You want to know what types of relationships he has had, what his attitudes about them are—if he's jaded, broken, bitter, a blamer, a shit talker, or angry. You also want to know why those relationships ended and what he learned from them—whether he is able to look back with a removed perspective and take ownership of his role in their problems or whether he finds himself totally blameless and faultless, both of which are revealing in themselves. Is he jaded—thinking that all women are conniving bitches and out to get him? Is he too fresh out of his relationship and still very broken? Are his walls up, protecting his heart? Is he open to loving again? Does everything bad always happen to him at no fault of his own? Does he talk trash about his exes in a nasty and aggressive manner? What made him fall for her and love her in the first place? How did the relationship start? Why and how did the relationship end? There is so much that can revealed about a person by tapping into pain points like failed relationships. If you want to get a guy raw and open and emotionally present, get him to talk about his ex. Ask questions. Let him talk. But know when to stop so that you don't cross the line from gathering information to prying. Try to upswing the conversation (that "U" formation), bringing the energy back up to a positive place by asking him what he learned and how he is an even more amazing person now because of the experience.

DON'T sound jaded, broken, bitter, or angry.

Why? You may have been hurt, hurt others, made gigantic mistakes, been totally screwed over; you may have even had a mangled heart and a messed up mind for a time. But that's not you anymore. You healed, picked up the pieces, and put yourself back together stronger and better than ever before. The you that you are today is no longer reeling in pain and bitterness. You are reveling in excitement for the next chapter!

DON'T talk as though you're still in love with him.

Why? It's a turnoff, plain and simple. The way you talk about your ex should be balanced. No dreamy or watery eyes. You're over him and ready for something fresh and wonderful and new!

DON'T go into things that no guy wants to hear about . . . ever—your sex life!

Why? I don't care how extraordinary, crazy, bizarre, awful, or simply perfect your sex life was with your ex; don't talk about it. Ever.

DON'T mention things that you wouldn't want to get back to your ex.

Why? You don't know who this guy knows, who he talks to, or who he *will* talk to about what you tell him about your ex. If this date ends up not being the end-all, be-all and you put some serious shit out there about your ex, your date could easily go off and blab about what you told him. Make a decision *before* your date about where your line is. This way you are in control of how much you reveal. He, however, isn't likely expecting you to extract the ex-talk out of him, so he could very well tell you more and go deeper than you—and that's fine. You have a line, and you aren't crossing it until you truly have established trust with this guy. If, for a second, you question whether or not you should reveal something, the asnswer is NO.

DON'T continue the ex conversation for more than twenty minutes—combined.

Why? While you learned from the past, you aren't living in it. You are living in the present and looking to move into a future—maybe with *this* new guy. This isn't a therapy session. If he's the one who keeps going on and on about his ex, pull him out of it and back into the present by asking him what he learned, how he's different or better, or what he will do or look for this time around. Or just change the subject by bringing up a thread of an element that he mentioned in a story, for example, "You mentioned that you went skiing in Switzerland. I love to ski!" Then continue telling a story about your last ski trip.

When it comes to ex-talk, it's not about dwelling in the past. The purpose is to learn more about him, to reveal more about yourself, to be on the lookout for red flags, and hopefully to connect on a deeper, more authentic level.

HOW DO YOU INITIATE THIS LINE OF CONVERSATION? EASY!

Here are some generic intro lines that can start the ex-talk:

- "You seem like a pretty amazing guy. What girl let you go so that I got to go out with you tonight?"

- "It's amazing how much we learn from past relationships. I know I have made a ton of mistakes in the past. Even from breakups that left me brokenhearted, I still was able to extract the good and have takeaway that made me better and stronger and more ready this time around. What did you learn in your last relationship?"

- "How has your online dating experience been? I've actually enjoyed it. It has been great to meet different people with varied backgrounds and life experience. It has also helped me to better understand what I really need in a relationship. What about you? What made you go online in the first place?"

- "Wow, I can't believe you're (X age) and still single. What's wrong with you?"

- "Really, you cheated on your last girlfriend? What an asshole! Why would you do that?"

- "Really, your last girlfriend cheated on you? What were you doing wrong that made her want to stray?"

Put him down and you'll wall him up. Ask questions but don't interrogate. Be sensitive to his hardships, but don't be his mother. Don't judge him (at least not verbally). If you think he's a dick, keep it to yourself and just never go out with him again. Let him talk, but don't let it become a therapy session. Make sure to have a two-way conversation—which includes both speaking and asking.

FRIEND ZONE AND BOOTY CALLS:
HOW TO AVOID THEM

These two stories have the type of excitement and passion you might find in the movies. But they are pages out of my life. They may start similarly, but they end differently: one in a relationship and the other as sex buddies.

We were introduced during a get-together at a super hip and sexy pool-side bar in LA, and we instantly hit it off. From the moment he entered our area, I demanded that he sit next to me. But, with no spare chair, I allowed him to share mine. Apparently he was some hotshot business guy and the boss of one of the girls' boyfriends, so someone promptly brought him his own seat. Despite being surrounded by a half-dozen friends, we honed in on each other and fell into witty and flirty banter. An hour or so into the conversation, we both wanted yet another drink and the service wasn't up to par for him, so, instead of waiting for the overwhelmed server to return to our group, we decided to go inside and order from the bar.

It was loud, so we spoke close, our lips mere inches apart. And then he kissed me. It was the kind of kiss that literally makes you dizzy, so I wrapped my arms around him as his tongue twisted around mine. "Get a room!" yelled a sickened bystander, which forced us to sort of come to the realization that our kiss was more than a mere moment in time. We found a couple of chairs in a corner and decided not to rejoin the group out-side, as we continued our too-comfortable make-out session. Last call was announced, and we spotted our friends leaving, including my guy's ride. We hurried over and his friend said, "Have fun! Laurel, I assume you can bring him back to my place tomorrow?" Having had too much to drink and completely entranced by the intensity of the chemical attraction that drew me to him, I said, "Sure!" and then realized, "Holy shit, this guy is coming home with me!" We got into a cab and went back to my place. And that was only the beginning of our night. . . .

The next morning we went out to breakfast, where he announced that he had to head to the airport in a few hours to go home. He had meetings the next afternoon. "Nope!" I flirtatiously retorted. "You need to take me on a proper date to make up for last night." He smiled and explained that he really had to head back. He never missed Monday meetings. "But if you go back, you might miss having another experience like last night with me again," I responded with a sweet sideways smile. He proceeded to go through his phone and type out several e-mails. A few minutes later he said that he was staying until tomorrow. Since he hadn't spent much time in LA, I took him to a few of my favorite spots. We talked a lot and got to know each other, then went out to a fun sushi dinner. As the evening came to an end and we were on our way back home to my house, he said that he had to see me again and wanted to fly me to New York the following weekend. I jokingly said that I was very busy and that he would have to fly me first class if I was to go. He agreed and said it would be taken care of when he returned home. The next morning I drove him to the airport and told him to text me when he landed. . . .

So what do you think? Relationship or sex buddy?

Well, he texted me when he arrived home, and the following day he called, asking whether I was still interested in meeting him in New York. When I responded, "Yes!" a few hours later my itinerary arrived in my e-mail. First class. We continued to have weekend dates in different places—his home and other cities he traveled to for business—and within six months I moved out of LA and in with him. We were together for two and a half years. How did I transform what could have been a one night fling into a full-blown relationship? I asked for what I wanted—in a sweet and flirtatious way—because I knew I deserved it. I showed him that I thought highly of myself, and so should he. Sure, he was wealthy, good-looking, and young, and he probably could have gotten almost any woman he wanted. But that didn't intimidate me. Could it have gone another way? Absolutely. The whole thing was a very careful dance rooted in self-confidence.

And now for story two . . .

When that last relationship ended, I was a wreck. He was a very opinionated man, and somehow I lost my way with him. And I lost myself. But that's another story. So, after we broke up and I moved back to LA, it took me some time to rebuild my self-esteem. I had a hard time socializing and hardly knew how to have a conversation because I no longer truly knew who I was. I didn't even look like myself. A few months before I had ended the relationship, I took out my need for change on my hair in an attempt to avoid what I really needed to do—break up. So I cut my nipple-length hair, transforming it into a jawline bob, then dyed it from golden to dark chocolate brown. The day I returned to LA, I went back to blonde, but it was still short, and I still didn't recognize me in the mirror. Extensions quickly solved that, returning my hair to its long blonde state in a matter of hours.

After several weeks of being a hermit, refusing to emerge from the safety of my new home, a friend suggested that I finally get out of my funk and go with her to a *Goldfinger*-themed holiday party. It was my first real outing since the breakup. Feeling more like a wallflower than a *Goldfinger*-infused seductress, I affixed myself to my girlfriend's hip and spoke only when spoken to. And then this strikingly hot guy with a big warm smile and perfectly messed-up hair walked in. Clearly he was "somebody," and everyone was vying for his attention, including my friend, who seemed to actually know him. She introduced us, and I held out my sweaty hand and said hi. And that was about it. For the next few hours, I attempted to make some sort of interesting conversation with the many people my friend knew, but I couldn't help continuously glancing over at that guy. And occasionally I saw him reciprocating as we accidentally made eye contact, which of course I instantly broke. Unable to leave without my preoccupied friend, I found a quiet spot in another room and hid out on a sofa pretending to check my phone. And then I felt a leg press up beside mine. It was him. He asked what I did for a living, and I told him that I was a writer. He said that he wrote music too, but he was really a singer and suggested that maybe I had heard of some of his stuff. Used to the bullshitters in LA, I assumed he was just a big talker, but I actually really enjoyed our conversation. We discussed music and the art of writing and how we found inspiration and what it felt like to craft the perfect sentence. It was thrilling and I was taken by him. Hours passed, and my friend came over to say that she was going home and asked him if he wouldn't mind dropping me off because clearly we were in the midst of conversation. He said that he didn't mind at all. For a moment my thoughts wandered back to the bar with my ex as I recalled the relationship that resulted from a similar situation almost three years before. This could be the start of something great! After a little while we decided it was time to go. The party was winding down, and there was no reason to stick around. We went out to his car and proceeded to make out for about an hour. The windows were fully steamed—a good thing considering that passersby would have certainly enjoyed the very X-rated show! Then he dropped me off at home.

The next day I texted to say that I had fun and we should do that again sometime. Turned out he really was a pretty well-known singer/ songwriter. And yes, I actually used to love one of his songs. Intimidated and feeling undeserving of his attention, I jumped at the chance to see him again when he asked if I wanted to hang out after a dinner that he had to go to. Instead of saying that I would rather wait for another night when he could take me to dinner (instead of having me for dessert), I took what I felt I could get and degraded myself to an after-dinner booty call. The next morning I felt like shit about it. A week or so later he again texted to ask me out for a late-night "drink." I said no. I had regained an understanding of my worth and wasn't going to sell myself short again. When I started demanding better, I got it. Soon we became friends—not with benefits. We resumed that conversation that we first had at the party as I elevated myself back up and regained his respect as a writer with a brain, not just a fun girl with a body.

Could that night have turned out differently? Probably. But I lost control when I forgot my value, neglected to set my limits and standards, and effectively said that I wasn't worth more than booty-call status. Yet another mistake-based lesson learned. You're welcome.

* * *

You don't want to be deemed a friend when you can't stop thinking about swapping spit. You don't want to be just a sex buddy when you imagine your fingers entangled, strolling down the street like two peas in the perfect-relationship pod. Both situations are frustrating, even emotionally painful. And both are equally easy to slip into but difficult to maneuver out of.

It's all about setting a precedent from the onset. Sure, friends *can* turn into lovers and sex buddies *might* evolve into more, but you will up your chances of getting what you want out of the relationship if you're clear with your intentions from the very beginning—the first date.

FRIEND ZONE

Are you that girl who, no matter what you do or say, no matter how exactly you follow the rules (or the nonrules) of dating engagement, no matter how clear you think you're being that you are interested in this guy—even if you do some making out on the first date—somehow you still end up as just friends? You might be beautiful, smart, have an amazing career and a drool-worthy body . . . you're seemingly the total package and you *still* are placed in the friend zone! But this doesn't just happen once; it happens repeatedly. If this keeps happening, it's not him—it's you.

So what are you doing wrong, when everything you do seems to be so by-the-book right? Here are several mistakes that you might be making, each of which could land you in the friend zone.

You don't make him work for it or pay for it. Think about how he is with his career. The more effort he puts into his career and the more money he makes, the more he is worth to the company, and the more he values his job. Same goes for dating. If a man has to put effort into the relationship and spend some money, he automatically equates you with value. He is paying for dinner. I already talked about this, but since it's important, I thought I should repeat it.

You are fun, sweet, family oriented, successful, pretty, and smart . . . and that's it. You talk about vacations, music, books, movies, culture, and a little bit about work, but you're careful not to address hot topics or dive into anything too personal. After all, you don't want to scare him off by making him tap into unpleasant emotions, you think. Staying light is better and more fun too, you say. But that's exactly the problem! Didn't you read the section about being real and getting raw? Most guys have dated plenty of "fun, pretty, sweet" girls. If that's all you are, you're forgettable. Forgettable! That's the last thing you want to be. If you want to stand out, then be your perfectly unique self. Think about it this way: What is it that you most love about those who are closest to you? That they are pretty? Smart? Perfect? Sweet? Sure those are nice, but what you really love, what makes them stick in your heart, are their quirks, their vulnerabilities, the things that make them human. Why do you hide those things that make you most lovable?

You lead with your head and you aren't intriguing. Sure, you're smart and successful. You may even be beautiful with a banging body. But you are rigid and you aren't sexy! You don't know how to flirt. You don't intrigue him and make him want to know more. You don't make him have this sense that you have lots of secrets, and maybe even a dirty side, hidden behind that ideal exterior—and that's what he really wants to explore. Being intriguing and sexy doesn't mean being slutty. It's about the little things: the side glance, the secret smile, the little touches, the flirtatious and slightly (but not overtly) sexy comments and texts: it's about the X Appeal. It might feel weird to you at first. You might not be comfortable "being that person." And that's okay. It's like a muscle that you need to strengthen. At first you might in fact act silly or awkward or even make a fool out of yourself. But once you let go of your rigidity and you soften into the feminine, you will get it. The section on "How to Walk into a Room and Own It" can help.

You are paper-perfect. And that's about it. You aren't real. You aren't flawed. You haven't had to fight and overcome demons. You have "Stepford Wife" written all over your face. What's missing? *You!* No one is that perfect. Everyone has nuances and weaknesses and quirks, and that's what makes us unique and relatable and lovable. Pull the stick out of your ass and be real. I know it can be scary to let your guard down. You might not even know why you have it up there so high. Something may have happened in your childhood that forced you to erect a shield as protection. Address it. Dig deep and try to figure out what it is that is keeping you so uptight and not allowing you to exhale. It's okay. You don't have to be perfect anymore. The U Dig Strategy in the "Get Unstuck" section can help.

You act like a buddy. You hang out at sports bars. You don't put effort into how you look. You don't mind paying for some things or going Dutch. You talk and act like a man. It's okay to share the same interests. It's okay if you are a huge sports fan. But remember that you are looking for a boyfriend, not a buddy. Be feminine—which doesn't necessarily mean girly. You can still be sexy and cheer on your favorite team.

You are too type A. Both you and he know how successful in business you are. And it's awesome that you are powerful and financially secure (maybe even financially superior to him), but soften up and lose the edge when you're with him. If you are a type-A control freak, then be in charge of letting go. Make the decision to be a little sweeter, a little softer, and little less assertive and aggressive. Be a little coy, a little vulnerable, a little more emotionally supple.

You think you're being sarcastic, but you're actually being a bitch. I know, you want to be witty and always have a comeback, and I agree! Those are both great talents when it comes to flirting. But there is a difference between sarcastic and bitchy, and it's too often confused—so much so that I would stay away from sarcasm altogether and stick with witty instead. Sarcastic folds into bitchy when you are putting him down, questioning his manhood, making him feel lesser in any way, or being cutting and jabbing. Witty, however, shows your whip-smarts, your range of knowledge and experience, and your quick-on-your-feet thinking. It's not rude, degrading, snobby, or elitist. Be careful with your word choice and snappy commentary, particularly over text and e-mail, where tone is left out of the very important sarcasm equation. Before you say something sarcastic, first think about how it is going to come out and how you would feel if he said that to you.

You're too easygoing. You don't require dates. You just kind of hang out. While being easy might seem like a turn-on, guys actually do enjoy a little bit of the chase. They are turned on by putting effort into the date. If he has to think about what to do and where to take you, that means that you are in his mind as he is making the plan, and he is then more invested in the date and how much you like it. It's also the anticipation all day that will get him excited about the activity and in turn about you.

BOOTY CALL / SEX BUDDY

Sleeping with him too soon doesn't automatically doom you to sex buddy status. It's more about attitude than actions. That said, just because you say, do, and carry the confidence needed to set your standard as girlfriend material and not a booty call doesn't mean that you will automatically obtain that status. You can't control him. You can only control yourself. While you might be in the ideal head, heart, and financial space to be in a relationship, that doesn't mean he's there too. If you ask the prequalifying questions that shed light on his current mental and emotional state, then you have the power to make decisions based on his responses. If you choose to be available to the guy and exploit your worth for his every whim without requiring him to treat you with the high-value respect that you deserve, you have to be cognizant of the possible repercussions. If you don't view yourself as worthy—as reflected in your attitude and expectations—why would he?

On a date, what do you do to establish yourself as a high-value and sexy woman?

Be feminine and flirty, but strong and confident.

Be on-purpose with your core values and your dating purpose. Just having those in your mind will naturally allow you to act on-purpose even without trying.

Remember your value and your intentions.

Be interesting and interested. You have something to contribute to the conversation and, if you choose to move forward with this relationship, you have something to contribute to his life.

Be that chick! Make him feel like he is lucky to be out with you. He wouldn't want to do anything to sabotage such luck. Sure, he may see how far he can push, but set your limits and sweetly let him know that there is no pushing past them.

He pays the check. Period. This is a date, not a freebie. You pay for things that are worthwhile. And your time and presence are worthwhile.

He's just a guy. Make him feel good about himself. But be sure to insert a few of your kickass qualities, too. Even if he's smarter, wealthier, or better looking than you and you secretly think you're not good enough for him—get over it! He's just a guy, and you are an awesome woman who is so worthy of him. In fact, is he worthy of you?

Get raw. Be real, dig deep, show that quirky and human side of you that makes you memorable while simultaneously creating an environment of trust that makes him feel safe to open up too.

Remember that you aren't auditioning for him. You are both feeling each other out and trying to decide whether you are right for each other. He needs to impress you just as much as you need to impress him. This is a two-way street. Stop trying to impress him and instead simply be your fabulous self.

Sexy, sultry, sassy, trashy, a challenge, witty, biting, spontaneous, wild, and fun . . . may make him interested for now, but that girl doesn't often get him to go down on bended knee. Sexy, pretty, intriguing, interesting, challenging (different than a challenge), confident, wise, respectful, respectable, worthy, fun, comforting, sweet, and quirky are what maintains a man's interest.

IF YOU'RE NOT INTERESTED, HE'S CRAZY ABOUT YOU—IF YOU *ARE*, HE'S NOT

This is one of the most common things I hear from clients. It's something that is agonized about, debated, and overanalyzed. But really the reason for this unequal level of interest is simple: when it doesn't matter you act more like yourself, plus you're aloof. When it does matter you either act how you think you should act or how you think he wants you to act, or you have no idea how to act so you're awkward, shut down, overly excited, always available, shy, quiet, bitchy, sarcastic, over the top, dumbed down, insecure, all in, guarded, pessimistic, needy, anxious, avoidant, etc.

If you consistently fall into this zone, you've got to do your best to *be yourself* and remember: he's just a guy. Sure he's hot, rich, successful, smart, respected, or he just has that chemical click that you *need*; but let's put things into perspective here—*he is just a guy*. And he sure as hell is not perfect, regardless of how *perfect* a few key elements may seem to be about him. Don't let your trancelike state blind you into thinking he's any better than he actually is. He is flawed. He has quirks that will eventually aggravate the hell out of you. Rate each of his traits equally and appropriately. For example, if he's really hot, does it make sense to rank looks on the same level as emotional availability when it comes to what's actually important in a relationship? And sure—he's rich, but when compared to kindness, communication, or valuing you as an equal partner, what holds up to be more of a relationship-enduring quality?

Once you put things into perspective and you realize that you have a lot to bring to the table and that he's actually lucky to be with you, suddenly you have taken the control back, and you will be able to draw him in instead of push him away. Knowing and being confident in your worth and contribution to this relationship comes from a combination of your purpose and your core values.

ATTITUDE OF ABUNDANCE

Even if you aren't dating several guys and you really don't have any other viable prospects, you still need to have an attitude of abundance, the operative word being "attitude." This is about putting off the energy that, although you think this guy is fantastic and you honestly do hope it works with him, there truly are plenty of fish in the sea, and you can easily pull in another guy just as great or better if need be. An attitude of abundance is an attitude of confidence. It's knowing that you are a valuable commodity. Yes—you are worth something. A lot actually! As is your time and the energy that you put into being on this date. To clarify: an attitude of abundance is not an attitude of arrogance. This isn't about being a snob or treating him like he's unimportant. It's about knowing your worth. *And that's sexy.*

THE MAKE OR BREAK: VACATION DATE

You're done playing the field. You have decided to X out the rest and focus your attention on one fabulous guy who seems to have serious potential. This guy is different from the others. You have great chemistry, he makes you laugh, your conversations are engaging, so you agree to be exclusive and cut the line with all of the other guys you were pursuing. Still, you have been down this road before, and as soon as the façade is dropped and he reveals his real side, suddenly this match seems less made in heaven and more made in momentary fantasy. So, put it to the test. Instead of wasting time waiting until the other shoe drops or he lets down his guard and exposes his true colors, create an environment that encourages transparency—one that isn't about being on all the time but is instead about being real. Go on vacation. You learn *a lot* about a person when traveling together:

- What are his habits?

- How high-maintenance is he?

- How long does it take him to get ready?

- Is he moody in the morning?

- If things don't go his way, does he freak out?

- How does he treat servers, housekeepers, bellhops?

- Does he have a similar dating purpose?

- Does he get easily annoyed?

- Is he adventurous?

- Do you have a similar rhythm?

- Do you have similar styles of communication?

- Is he cheap?

- Do you have things to talk about?

- Is he emotionally supportive and nurturing if you get scared?

- Can he go with the flow?

- Do you balance each other out?

I call it a make or a break. Go out of town together, and you'll immediately know whether this relationship has potential (if it's a make) or not (if it's a break). This isn't about having sex. If you're not there yet—no problem! Sleep in separate beds, or rooms, even! This is about spending extended time together and getting to know each other on a level that usually takes months to experience.

So where do you go? Far enough away so you can remove yourself from your daily life, giving you the opportunity to truly focus on each other. However, you don't want to go so far that, if it's a break, the trip home is loooong and uncomfortable.

The goal is to drop your guard and really be yourselves. By the end of the trip, you'll know if it's a make or a break. And if it's a make, you'll have so much more experience together that will enrich your relationship right off the bat, helping to create a more fortified foundation. If it's a break, well, at least you found out sooner rather than later so you don't have to waste any more time.

CHAPTER 4

How to Keep Him . . . and Sex

THE DANGER OF HAVING SUCH POWER OVER MEN

Before I continue to reveal my secrets to get a man to fall head-over-heels, obsessively, you're-the-one in love with you—fast, I have to do the responsible thing and warn you that wielding this type of power can also be dangerous. What you are creating is kind of like microwaved love—fast love formed from the inside out. But that doesn't mean it will be easy. You will endure bumps in the road and emotional flexes and fluxes that come when two fully formed people fold together in the creation of a relationship. You won't always be in sync; your opinions and lifestyles won't always align, and neither will your moods or levels of connection and emotional progress. And that's okay. Be aware that those phases may come faster as you quickly experience intense feelings that might feel like a roller coaster, as they almost pile up on top of each other.

What are these phases? I view relationships like a wedding cake with multiple tiers. Each tier is another level of the relationship. As you go up a tier, you are getting closer to the top. It's exciting! Things are great! And then you move in along the top of the tier toward the center during moments that might be tough or confusing. Get through those tough moments, and you are actually moving closer together. And then you get to fly high again as you zoom up the side of another tier! Repeat, repeat, repeat. Here's what you will likely experience:

WEDDING CAKE LOVE

HEART CONNECTION

What you're experiencing: Your heart has been tapped. You start at the bottom of the wedding cake. Everything is just dandy, and your relationship flies straight up the first tier. Your partner seems like your ideal match! You love being together and you feel like you will be happy forever! You finally found your one!

What to do: In this time, you need to be honest about your needs, and set boundaries and expectations. It's all moving so fast, but you have to maintain control and create a foundation that prepares you for the next phase.

REALITY

What you're experiencing: Now you are going across the bottom tier of the cake, and you feel like you are plateauing. You start to see that you're not always in sync. Issues may come up. Real life starts to get in the way. You spent so much time making him the priority that you might feel behind in work or that you've been neglecting friends. You start to pull back a little. You show real sides of you while noticing the not-so-perfect sides of him, too. In the heart connection phase, you were always in the mood, but now you're not. Your heart doesn't always race when he is on his way to pick you up. You don't get as turned on by his touch. Little things start to irk you, and you begin to feel disillusioned and start to question why you were so crazy about him in the first place. Though it may not feel like it, you are actually coming toward each other along the top of the tier, getting closer with each hardship.

What to do: Communicate. Don't shut down or run away. Don't suddenly load up your life with excuses as to why you can't see him. Remind yourself why you were crazy about him in the first place. Make time for him, but slowly back off a bit and take time for yourself. It's natural for men to start to pull back a bit during the reality phase. And it's not because he is no longer interested. It's because his life and priorities shifted to fit you into it, and suddenly he is experiencing the result of that shift. He may also feel the awkwardness of his heart opening—which can be confusing for someone who hasn't really *felt* for quite a while. As he begins to feel for you, he could simultaneously experience a touch of fear, which is often the fear of being out of control. Don't get frantic. Don't start questioning him. Don't act insecure. One of the things he likes most about you is how confident you are. Show him otherwise, and this pull-back period could be the end of your relationship. Instead, give each other a little space and take the freed-up time to explore your interests and expand your life.

REAL CONNECTION

What you're experiencing: Enjoy the thrill of whizzing up the side of another tier! You got through the reality phase together, and you found that you actually love and like him much more than before. You saw the real him, and he saw the real you, and he's still here and you are too! You are closer now because you experienced and overcame difficulty together. Your relationship is now more mature, accepting, and understanding. You are feeling real love, as opposed to the heart connection infatuation that you felt before.

What to do: Enjoy the deeper connection and explore your interests together. Now is the time to have more substantive time together. Enjoy day dates where you have the opportunity to feel what it's like to just live together. By "live together," I don't mean that you are moving in together, but you are experiencing what a shared life feels like. Do mundane things like going to the farmer's market, running errands, and just being with each other in real, daily life situations.

Warning: Just because you have ascended to a level of comfort doesn't mean that you can get so comfortable as to stop putting effort into the relationship. You have to continue to try—to flirt, get dressed up, maintain your appearance and attitude. As comfortable as you may feel, don't stop being that sexy, feminine woman who he fell in love with. Don't degrade his view of you by showing the gross—albeit real—sides of you. What I mean is that you shouldn't start going to the bathroom in front of him, farting, "forgetting" to shave, wearing "period" panties, picking your nose, or other unattractive things. You can be comfortable, have old married couple routines, let your guard down, enjoy wearing cozy sweats instead of sexy shorts while lounging around, and *still* make an effort.

REFLECTION

What you're experiencing: He has seen you during your not-so-pretty moments. He loves you without makeup and finds your authentic self even more appealing than the façade you put on when out in public. Your "secret" side, the side of you that isn't perfect, is his favorite side because no one else gets to see it but him. You have been accepted for the real you, which makes you feel safe and trusting. Your heart is opening more completely than it has in a long time.

Warning #1: Within that comfort, openness, and letting your guard down, you may suddenly start to experience real insecurities. Old fears and weaknesses start to show themselves again. You are dreaming about ex-boyfriends, and you don't understand why *now*—now that you are happy and found someone fantastic? I'll tell you why: it's because you feel safe again. With that feeling of safety, you are actually *feeling* again. Your heart has unnumbed. The ice has melted. You are exploring emotional crevices that you haven't experienced in a long time. And within those crevices hide some unresolved feelings, like tar bubbling up from your core. This doesn't mean that he is just like all the others or even that he is the reason you are feeling this way. It's your past that just needs to be worked through in order to be worked out of your system. You're going along the top of a tier again, and even though it doesn't feel like it right now, you are actually working your way closer to each other.

What to do: Take some time for you. This doesn't mean that you need to take a break from the relationship, but it might make sense for you to do some healing. You may feel like you need to hibernate. And that's okay. Don't push past the pain and maintain your regular routines if you truly aren't feeling it, because you could end up feeling annoyed or overwhelmed as you start to shut down and turn cold fast. Instead, be honest with your partner. Let him know that some old stuff is bubbling up. It's not anything that he did wrong; it's actually because he's so right. Tell him that because you have, for the first time in a long time, opened your heart again, you are experiencing some residual fears and insecurities. This is an opportunity to bring your communication to a new level of closeness.

Warning #2: If either of you starts to feel turned off or shut down, don't freak out. It's actually oddly normal to go through this turmoil during times when you are feeling closest. This can happen after a fantastic vacation or a date that results in turning it up a notch as your commitment to each other increases. Again, this doesn't mean that you are all of the sudden over it. You are simply being triggered by old habits, pain points, and lingering fears. If he is the one going through this, you might feel shut out, or you could take on the burden of his annoyance, anger, sabotaging, or silence. You probably feel powerless, scared, or frantic. Don't emotionally detach or do the opposite—don't get needy. Now is the time to communicate. Be empathetic and understanding of yourself and him. Allow for space, but keep up the connection and you will just continue getting closer, and soon you will be enjoying the feeling of propelling up the next tier. If the issues are deep and intense, it might make sense to seek a therapist who can help to exorcise them.

What you're experiencing: Now that the old pain has been excavated and the emotional blocks have been pulled down, you have even more room for the new and healthy feelings of love for this man who is wonderful to you. You can truly open and share your heart. Enjoy the closeness that comes from complete trust and transparency.

What to do: Continue to put effort into your relationship. This is not the time to get lazy or take advantage of your relationship. Yes, routines are important, but so is maintaining that spark. Remember to do the little things that make each other feel like a priority, even amidst a crazy busy day.

Warning #1: Until you have experienced all tiers of the cake, don't get engaged.

Warning #2: Know that you may repeat tiers. Give yourself permission to make mistakes. Be patient. You are creating new patterns, and sometimes you can't help but slip up. What's important to remember is that it doesn't matter how many times you fall; it matters how many times you get back up again.

Warning #3: You or he may miss the thrill of the initial chase. Everything feels easy now. You don't always have to have butterflies. And that's okay. Embrace how great comfort and consistency feel. If you or he truly needs that old thrill, this is where fantasy, spontaneity, even role play can come in. Entice those butterflies to flutter again by flirting with each other and bringing back a level of mystery and fun, within the comfort and safety of your solid relationship.

WHEN SHOULD YOU HAVE SEX?

First date, fifth date, ninety days, in a serious committed relationship, on your wedding night? My honest opinion as to when you should have sex is—it doesn't matter. No, I'm not saying that when you have sex doesn't matter. I'm saying that *my* opinion as to when *you* should have sex doesn't matter. The only opinion that matters is yours.

Sex is a personal and private matter and not something that someone else can dictate—that someone else includes me, your best friend, your mom, your mentor, or the person you are going to have sex with. Only you can make the decision as to when the time is right for you. There are couples who have sex on the first date and end up in totally healthy, enduring relationships that lead to happy and fulfilling marriages, just as there are people who have sex on the first date and never speak again, just as there are couples who waited until they were in a committed relationship and broke up after a few months, just as there are couples who don't have sex and don't go beyond date eight. So what's the rhyme and reason? There isn't one. Here are the facts:

- Most first dates don't turn into relationships.

- Having sex once in a committed relationship doesn't guarantee that you'll stay together.

- Having sex is an emotional and physical act that can help further bond your connection and simultaneously be a lot of fun.

Want to have sex on the first date? Go ahead if that's what you want. But here's the one important thing to keep in mind *if* you want to up your chances of being respected after, having the sex turn into a relationship, and not beating yourself up for doing it: have emotional intimacy *before* physical intimacy. If you prequalified effectively first, you've already started building that emotionally intimate relationship.

Here are the dos and don'ts when it comes to first-date (or any date) sex:

BE SAFE!

Have protected sex. Being on the pill doesn't count. Carry condoms and use them. It's not just the guy's responsibility to be responsible.

Protect yourself emotionally. Communicate your honest expectations before the deed is done, and you are less likely to be emotionally distraught after.

COMMUNICATE!

Prequalify him first. Assuming that you thoroughly prequalified him before going on the first date, you actually should know each other pretty well and you may already have created the foundation for a real and substantive relationship.

Open your mouth before you open your legs. If you are comfortable enough to open your legs, open your mouth first. Communicate. Talk about your dating purpose so you can gauge whether you're on the same page.

Get raw. Sex isn't just about fucking. It's about being vulnerable and open and raw. If you're not comfortable being raw, then you aren't ready to have sex—regardless of your purpose.

BE HONEST AND TRUE TO YOU!

Don't feel pressured. *Only* have sex if *you* really want to have sex. It's your decision.

Deep emotional connection or not, take it for what it is—sex. It's physical and emotional pleasure. It's fun. It's relaxing and revitalizing. It doesn't have to be a big thing. But if you make a big thing out of it, it will be.

No regrets. Don't destroy yourself, beat yourself up, demonize yourself, or trash-talk yourself after. If you're going to regret it, don't do it! If you are questioning whether you should do it and you feel like you should stop it—don't have sex!

HAVE FUN!

Have fun and let go! If you're not going to be there emotionally, don't go there physically. Either fully commit on to the act or save it for later. Make a decision—which means to decide yes or no, not "I don't know, I guess."

If it's bad, don't freak out. Sex with a new partner isn't always great. That doesn't mean that he or you are bad in bed. You may have different styles. With practice (and communication—which I discuss later), your styles will fold together, and you *will* find your rhythm.

UNDERSTAND THE EXPECTATIONS

Just because you had sex doesn't mean you are in a relationship. It also doesn't mean that he wants a relationship with you. Don't make it so weighty. Don't immediately turn needy or clingy after. If you know that you normally become attached after you have sex with a guy—don't have sex on the first date! Wait until you are in a committed, monogamous relationship.

Just because you had sex on the first date doesn't mean that you're a slut. You're a sensual person. And that's fine. You just need to realize and be okay with the fact that you could be racking up lots of guys under your belt. If you're going to look down on yourself for it, then absolutely do not do it.

Do not use sex to try to get him to want you. That's not the purpose. This isn't about manipulation or games.

Do not open up your legs as an alternative to opening up your heart. That's where having sex can become emotionally dangerous. If you can't be present, in the moment, and emotionally available, don't do it.

If you are looking for emotional validation by having sex, don't do it.

If you are the person who shuts down during sex, who turns on your body and turns off your mind as your thoughts drift somewhere else in order to satisfy him but save yourself—don't do it! You have issues that you need to clear first (in the "Get Unstuck" section). Do not use your body as escapism from your mind.

If you're doing it for him, *don't do it!* Sex is an act between two people and for two people.

If you think, "I might as well," don't do it! You should want to have sex because you are feeling so connected and sexy and you want to dig deeper into his body and mind!

THERE ARE ALSO DANGERS
OF *WAITING* TO HAVE SEX

I'm not saying that waiting to have sex until monogamy is stupid. I'm simply saying it's your decision. In fact, it is possible to have an amazing first date and have *the* conversation, mutually deciding that you're ready and be in a monogamous, committed relationship! However, if you are dating someone for a while and your romantic dinners are repeatedly followed by heavy make-out sessions but no sex, when you send the guy home with blue balls each and every time, unless you communicate your decision to abstain and what your threshold is, he might feel like you're

- teasing him

- playing a game

- a prude

- maybe bad in bed

- not really that interested

- aren't true to your feelings

- too controlled

This makes him feel

- frustrated—both physically and emotionally

- unattractive

- not good enough

- rejected

- not trusted

- not trusting

- emotionally disconnected

- over it

. . . In that order. Because of how he is feeling as a result of you not having sex with him, he might end the relationship. And it's not because you refuse to have sex with him. It's how he internalizes that denial. You can help the situation by having a conversation in which you communicate that you really are crazy about and turned on by him, but you want to wait until _____ (insert reason).

Sex can be an emotional glue. It can pull a guy even closer to you. If you're not comfortable going there yet, you still need emotional glue to keep him coming back for more. And that glue is in the form of getting raw, being vulnerable, showing him that you *do* trust him by opening up about your emotions and sharing the authentic side of you that you generally hide from public view. If you are shut down both emotionally and physically, be prepared to soon say bye-bye to this guy.

"I HATE MY BODY"... IS RUINING YOUR SEX LIFE

You're flawed. We all are. But do you truly want your guy to view your body as you do? Do you want him to be disgusted by your cellulite-dimpled thighs? Do you want him to fixate on the fact that one of your breasts is significantly smaller than the other? Do you want him to be grossed out by the flap of belly fat that bulges over your jeans? Or do you want him to view you—your body, your curves, and your skin—as beautiful and sexy? I get why you feel the need to point out your imperfections and insecurities. You want him to know that you're aware of them too. You want to address the issue instead of allowing it to remain the unsightly elephant in the room. Well, I'm going to let you in on a little secret: your man won't see your flaws unless you point them out.

Whether in the form of a question: "Do these jeans make my ass look fat?" "Do you think I'm gaining weight?" or a statement: "I am getting so much more cellulite." "My boobs are getting droopy." "I hate my cankles." Or *worse*—in response to a compliment that he pays you—**He:** "You look beautiful tonight. I love that dress on you." **You:** "No I don't. My ass looks fat. I feel so puffy and ugly." Don't point it out to your guy. Bitch about it to your mom, sister, best friend, therapist, or even me during a coaching session, just not to him! I mean really, do you *want* him to see your cellulite before he sees your smile? He fell in love with you for a reason. Don't taint it. Your guy wants to feel like he's with the hottest chick. He wants to feel like he scored! Why would you tell him otherwise? Why would you ruin his perception that you're super sexy just the way you are? Do you want him to start picking you apart—either in his mind or out loud to you? Do you want him to look at you and think, "Ew"? Is that how you want your guy to view you—really? Even if you think he's nuts (or lying) about how hot you are, let him go on thinking and talking about it. When he pays you a compliment, instead of shutting him down, simply look him in the eye with a sexy little smile and say thank you.

If you're insecure about your body and you show him, he will start to view you as you do, seeing your butt, stomach, and thighs through your eyes. And you really don't want that, do you? Considering how hard most women are on themselves, the last thing you want to do is shine a light on the flaws that you fixate on (but honestly most likely no one else even notices—and may even find beautiful!).

Chances are good that you're nastier to yourself than anyone else. In fact, you very well may treat yourself like your worst enemy, saying things to yourself that you would never allow someone else to say to a friend. Think about it: What is the internal dialogue that replays in your head? Is what you tell yourself true? Sure about that? Or are you lying to yourself? Why do you feel the need to spread those lies and taint the view that your guy has of you?

If you keep it up and you continue to reinforce how hideous your stomach is (in your head), how you lack ankle tapering, and the fact that your breasts are too small and you wish they were fuller and perkier like your friend Christine, pretty soon he will see it too.

So, instead, act confidently. Embrace your body regardless of its given (and aging) shape. Because that's the confident, sexy, strong, voluptuous (whatever your body type is) woman he first spotted from across the room and the person who he fell in love with. If there is something that you have truly always hated or that you have a hard time seeing change with the years, then do something about it. But that's another conversation and another book.

HOW TO BE THE BEST HE'S EVER HAD . . . IN BED

"You're the worst lay and head I have ever had." I don't think adding insult to injury was necessary when my boyfriend broke up with me. But some guys are just assholes. In the end, it was actually a good thing, though . . . because he was right. I was pretty bad. Very bad—the worst, according to him.

When my boyfriend told me I was bad in bed, I didn't take it lightly. In fact, I went into full-blown research mode. "No, I'm not going to be the girlfriend who sucked—and not in a good way. I want to be awesome. The best even! I want my next guy to not be able to get enough. I want him to love it so much that he can't even imagine cheating on me because he knows that no one will blow him as well as he gets it at home." I got over the insult and decided to take the comment as constructive criticism.

* * *

When it comes to sexual ability, there are three types of girls:

1. Bad

2. Fine

3. Amazing

The girls who are Bad and the girls who are Fine generally have no idea where they stand in this scheme. Why? Because no guy is going to tell the girl he's with that she gives bad or "just okay" head (unless he tells her upon breaking up with her like mine did). He might suggest sex instead, try to guide her with a few midact suggestions, or simply say that he's not really into blow jobs. But he won't say, "Look, you suck. Can you please figure out how to do a better job?"

Girls who are Good, however—they know it. Guys rave about how great they are. They tell them that it was the best head they've ever had, seem dumbfounded—"How do you do that to me?"—and might even prefer oral to actual sex.

But those girls generally aren't magically born with such talent. It's learned—through practice, guidance, paying attention to the guy's sounds and moves, and books. More than talent, guys can tell whether a woman is actually into it, which you have to be to give good head, by the way. You have to be focused; your mind can't wander elsewhere as you assume that your mouth, palm, fingers, and tongue will continue to perform in perfectly escalating harmony—because they won't. As soon as you get lazy and start to lose interest, so will he.

If you want to be amazing in bed, you've got to take notes. Ask him:

- "What did you most like?"
- "Did you like when I did that swirling trick with my tongue?"
- "Do you like it better when I use my hands too or just my mouth?"
- "Did you like when I cupped your balls in my hand?"
- "What can I do differently, better, stop doing all together?"

SO HOW DO YOU GO ABOUT ASKING FOR THESE NOTES?

Similar to how you aren't supposed to tell someone that they have a drinking problem when they are drunk or that they should seriously consider anger management classes when they are in a fit of rage, don't ask your guy how you did or how you're doing during or even immediately after sex. Instead, ask a few hours later, maybe at dinner, at breakfast, before falling asleep when just lying together in bed chatting at night, in a bath ... somewhere that you are both relaxed, open, focused on each other, and interested in communicating. Then say, "I really loved our sex today. It seemed like you liked it when I did _____. What else did you like? What about when I go down on you, what do you like the best that I do? Did you like it when I did that swirl with my tongue? What about when I started licking your balls? I want to make you feel good. What should I focus on more? What don't you like as much? I won't get upset, I really do want to know what you like and don't like."

See, you start with the good and ease into asking about the bad. The reason? He might think it's weird at first that you want to be criticized, not realizing that it can be constructive, that you won't get mad (DO NOT GET MAD AND USE THIS AGAINST HIM!), and that you truly would like his direction.

Here's the key: you have to take your ego out of it. You are asking to be told what you are bad at, what needs improvement, in addition to what you're good at. This is not about blowing smoke or fishing for compliments. If you can't handle the truth, don't ask for it. But if you don't ask for it, you're also limiting yourself. You're saying, "I'm okay not being great at this."

Beyond the quality of your blow job, notes are an opportunity to open communication with your significant other in a very honest and vulnerable way, which can seriously deepen your relationship and tighten your bond. Not to mention that you are showing him that you *really* want to please him (which he should appreciate), and that can only lead to better sex. And who doesn't want that?

CHAPTER 5

Love and (Eventually . . . Maybe) Marriage

SHOULD YOU GIVE YOUR MAN AN ULTIMATUM?

Give a guy an ultimatum, and his instinct may be to run for the hills before you can! Men are defensive creatures. They don't like being told that they have to do something "or else." *Instead of an ultimatum, it's time for you to start thinking realistically about what you truly want and need.*

Do not threaten to leave if he doesn't propose. This should never be a threat. This should be an honest conversation about what you want, need, and expect. "This is where I stand. Where do you stand? Are we on the same page?" Be aware of and ready for the potential repercussions. If he is not in the same place, you need to be okay with adjusting your expectations or making a change and moving out and on, even if that means breaking your own heart.

But before you get overly caught up in the proposal, ask yourself these questions:

- Is it just about the piece of paper?
- Do you want to be with him regardless of whether he is ready to get married right now?

- Where is the pressure to get married coming from? You? Society? Your friends? Your parents? Your insecurities? The need to nail him down?

- Why do you need to get married right now?

- How will your relationship change if you get married?

- If he is unwilling to get married, now or ever, will you be able to accept that? Or will you resent him, feel rejected, emotionally retreat, constantly question him, lose trust?

- Have you communicated both of your needs, expectations, limiting beliefs, relationship trajectory, and timelines honestly and without fear of consequence?

WHAT IS HE WAITING FOR?

If you have the conversation and he expresses that he wants to marry you, he wants to have kids with you . . . someday, he just isn't ready yet, then you need to think about that too. Is this truly the man you want to spend your life with? Are you really on a deadline? Or do you just want to speed things up a bit? Is it worth leaving him or having him leave you only to end up searching for your next guy for a year or four, then to end up in the same stagnant situation with someone who isn't as good for you, all the while knowing that, had you stayed with the other guy, by now you would be married, have a kid, and be living the life you always wanted. In fact, he just might be living that life with someone new, who isn't you . . . because you left.

If your guy is slow out of the gate, not ready to propose, not ready to take the next relationship step yet, it might be time to have a conversation—not a showdown, not a fight, not a sob fest—a conversation. Ask him, "When do you see yourself being ready?" "Is there something that you are not sure about yet?"

"IT'S NOT THE RIGHT TIME"

One response that many guys use is "It's not the right time." Well, what is the right time? Does he want to be settled first? What does "settled" mean, exactly? Does he have a certain annual income in mind before feeling ready to seal the deal? Is he too busy at work? Will that busy time pass, or is his career busy in general? If his career is too busy in general, that's just life. It will always be too busy. The time will never be exactly right. He just has to decide whether he wants to fit you into his life or have your presence as a side note. My parents got married immediately upon graduating from college. They got pregnant with me when my mom was an art teacher's aide at a local university and my dad was unemployed. Not exactly ideal timing. But guess what? They figured it out. My dad got his shit together. In fact, my coming into this world helped light a fire under his ass and propel him into the amazingly successful career that he has had.

WHAT'S THE RUSH?

I urge you to seriously think about why you want to get married so badly. Is it because your parents were married at your age and you want what they have? Or maybe your best friend or even your little sister just did the aisle walk. Maybe he's perfect on paper. Or perhaps he has potential and you think he is going to change, and everything will be better when you have a ring on your finger. It could be that you feel like it's just time. You have been together for two years, and it "makes sense" to take the next "natural" step. STOP. Do you want to spend the rest of your life with this man? Even if he stays the same jackass, lazy bum, work-obsessed, uninteresting, flirtatious, immature guy you really aren't that attracted to anymore? If you want to get married for the wrong reasons, you could find that your wedded hopes, expectations, dreams, fantasies don't actually come true.

If you know you want to marry this man, you are ready to take that next step now, and you're certain it's for the right reasons, here are two ways to have the conversation:

1. Be up-front about what you need, want, and expect.

If you want to get married within a year and get knocked up within two years, say it . . . if it's more than just a willy-nilly time frame, an actual "This is where I stand, this is the course I am on, are you with me?" Especially if you are at a time in your life when you feel like your window for having children is closing, being up-front with what you are looking for out of the relationship is essential. Be prepared for the reality that some men just won't commit. They have girlfriends for three years, then they feel like the relationship has run its course, and they jump ship. It's a pattern. Or maybe it's just you who he doesn't see a life with. He thinks you're great and he's really enjoying your relationship, but he doesn't see it going anywhere beyond where it is. You are on a ride that will end. The only question is, when? He knows that this relationship will not move into marriage. He will not be proposing. Although he wants kids, he does not want kids with you. You have a right to know that. So ask!

2. Don't ask for what you want, and you will get it.

The inclination of some guys is to do the opposite of what you push for. If you say you want him to propose by a certain date, while he may have previously had every intention to propose by that date, the mere fact that you required it has now made him decide to wait until after your due date. That is honestly childish and annoying but frustratingly common. Yes, some guys do need subtle hints in order to understand what you want. No guy wants to propose to someone who is going to turn him down. Let him know that you want it. Put it out there. Then shush up about it! Even subtle hints can feel like megaphone demands if redundantly expressed. The fact that you want to marry him isn't something that he likely will forget (despite his propensity to forget seemingly everything).

FLIRTING, LINGERIE, AND ORAL SEX:
PUT SOME EFFORT INTO YOUR RELATIONSHIP!

After one too many rumors and inappropriate glances to other women, I couldn't take it anymore. Why was my guy paying so much attention to every hot chick he saw?!

A few months after it was over, when we could both be honest without fear of repercussions, I asked him why the roving eye. He said that I stopped trying. I didn't make him feel sexy or wanted. I didn't flirt with him and give him naughty glances and say sexy things under my breath. He became … normal to me, like putting on socks with my running shoes. Just something you do. It wasn't exciting anymore. I had stopped putting effort into the relationship. Because I stopped trying, he stopped noticing me. Because he stopped noticing me, I got insecure. Because I got insecure, I started hiding my body from him and would no longer strut my confident, sexy self around the house naked just to tease him. Because I stopped strutting it, he stopped seeing me as a sexual being. Because he stopped seeing me as a sexual being and because he was still a *very* sexual being, he started paying more attention to other women. And the cycle spiraled out of control, we stopped having sex, our relationship fell off the tracks, we fought instead of fucked, and it was soon over.

* * *

There is a difference between work and effort. Work feels like it's something you have to do. It's an action with an end goal, a desired outcome of a paycheck or maybe a pat on the back. Effort, on the other hand, is done for a greater cause. That doesn't mean it will always be something that you want to do, but you know that the purpose is to maintain and deepen the connection between you and your guy. It is a journey.

Just the simple tweak of the word can change your attitude toward the energy required to maintain your relationship. Because, let me tell you right now, maintenance will be required. Living with and accommodating your man's schedule, needs, emotions, ups and downs, friends, and family will not always be easy, or even fun. In fact, sometimes it will suck. Sometimes you will look at him and think, "Why am I even bothering?!" Sometimes you will wonder what it was about him that made you fall for him in the first place. Sometimes you are going to be so over his quirks that you will have a hard time seeing anything good about him at all. And that's totally normal. But it doesn't have to be the norm. It's time to start putting effort back into your relationship.

EFFORT COMES IN MANY FORMS

- Little notes left in his jacket pocket to let him know that you love him
- Text messages in the middle of the day to tell him that you are thinking about him
- Making dinner to show him that you love to nurture him
- Stopping on your way home from work to pick up his dry cleaning so that he doesn't have to
- Having a calm conversation instead of erupting when he does something that upsets you
- Joining him at his cousin's wedding in North Carolina instead of heading out of town to that spa vacation with your girlfriends to show that you support his relationship with his extended family
- Going out of your way to make him feel like he is a priority even when you are slammed at work and hardly have time for yourself
- Maintaining your looks

This section is about maintaining your looks, and maybe even upping your game a bit too.

Remember at the beginning of your relationship, as you were shaving your legs and perfectly coiffing your pubes thinking, "I can't imagine ever not wanting to take the time to do this"?

What happened?

Sure he says he loves you even without makeup on, and that's sweet, but that doesn't mean you have permission to now wear makeup only when you get gussied up to go out with the girls!

Like women, men want to be wanted, they want to know that they are desired, they want to feel needed and loved, they want to see you trying. Just because you've moved in together or you've been going out for a year doesn't mean that suddenly he's blind. You can't just kill off the sexy girl that you once were—the one who seduced him—then wonder why the girl at the office wearing the short skirts and giving him attention is getting his attention back.

IS IT YOU OR IS IT HIM?

Maybe he just doesn't seem into you anymore. Maybe his eyes no longer linger on your ass as you shimmy out of your skirt after work. Maybe he hardly even seems to notice when you look good—and you know it because you put extra effort into it tonight! He used to find you sexy. You're sure of it. Aside from his normal guy wandering-eye tendency, you were the only one for him. Every time you got undressed, even if you weren't wearing the sexiest underwear (though you generally made an attempt), he couldn't help but stare, his lips slightly parted, his body completely frozen, his eyes focused on your curves. Now it seems like something else is always on his mind. He's distracted. When you have sex, which is now infrequent, it feels requisite, not hot.

But it's not just your sex life that has been affected by this shift. It's your self-esteem, your confidence, your own desire for sex. You don't feel sexy naked anymore. In fact, you feel just the opposite. The spark seems to have fizzled.

It's time to do something about it! It's time to turn your relationship around! Don't just sit there feeling insecure. It's time to show him that you've still got it–that you are a hot piece of ass. *His* hot piece of ass.

It all starts in your head. You prefer lounging in sweats at home, keeping your hair in an unkempt ponytail, and wearing your cozy mismatched bra and panties. Not anymore. Change your mind and your actions and your relationship will follow. Feel sexy and you will act sexy. Dress up, shave your legs, and adjust your attitude!

Flirt with him! Flirt with him when you go out. *Yes*, flirt! You may have already gotten him, but that doesn't mean that now you should just talk about the frustrating thing your mom said, how upset you are that you are gaining weight, that he forgot to put the toilet seat down again, or how stressed you are about money! Do you think that's sexy? Do you think that's going to make him want you? Do you think that kind of conversation is going to make you want him? No. It's not.

Wear your special-occasion lingerie. Like using your fancy silverware and china instead of keeping it stuffed in the back of the cabinet, it's time to start in wearing your sexy lingerie—often! Pull out the sex toys that have been in the back of your drawer since you bought them. Put on some makeup, do your hair, and make an effort. Any night, day, even breakfast can be a special occasion—if you make it one. I know, sexy lingerie isn't as comfortable as cotton panties. Well, having a lackluster relationship is worse. Believe me.

Don't forget the oral sex. Many men believe that once the ring is slipped on the finger, the oral sex goes out the door. Sadly, it's often true. But that's all about to change—with you! You might feel like you don't have time, it's faster to just have sex, your mouth hurts after, he never goes down on you, so why should you go down on him, or that it's just gross. Whatever the excuse, it's bullshit and you know it. Open your mouth and suck it up. And, yes I did intend that play on words.

Guys love oral sex *if* you are good at it. So how do you get good at it? Well, we already talked about that in the "How to Be the Best He's Ever Had . . . in Bed" section—ASK! Ask him what he likes. If you're insecure about your ability, tell him that you want him to guide you and tell you exactly how he likes it. The fact that you're putting in the effort and that you want to be great for him will turn him on. Then remember that practice makes perfect. But more than practicing to the point of perfecting the techniques, if you want to give good head, you've got to put some effort into enjoying it—even if you really don't. If your mind is wandering, if you're bored, if you're bouncing your head back and forth thinking "I wish he would just come already so I can go to bed!" he will know that you're not totally into it and, guess what—he will take even *longer* to get off. Yes, there are certain tried-and-true techniques that you should know to truly be the best he's ever had, and you can access them on my website: www.ScrewingTheRules.com/products.

MONTHLY CHECK-INS

It's easy to get out of sync, particularly if you are both busy and stressed. As life gets in the way, sometimes your relationship is pushed to the side, making you feel like you aren't a priority, resulting in sadness, resentment, distance, and sometimes the eventual end. And it's not because you're not into each other or even that you grew apart; it's just that your focus shifted, and your once super-important relationship took a backseat to seemingly everything else.

When you're out of touch with each other, you might not realize that there are seeds of hurt or annoyance that could potentially grow and bloom into full-blown issues if not addressed at the onset. Make it a priority to check in and talk about how you feel about the relationship once a month before those seeds have the opportunity to sprout. Plus, you bring your relationship out of the blur and back into focus. Talk about your connection, the things that he did for you that month that made you feel special and important, the things that he did that made you feel unimportant and hurt, address misunderstandings, bring up the things that you feel could be improved as well as strategies and solutions to make that happen. This isn't about fighting, bashing, or being defensive. You aren't coming in with a laundry list of little things that he did that pissed you off. Instead, you are coming together as a unit to talk about the ways you can strengthen your connection.

At the end of each month, scheduled on your calendar, check in with your guy. It doesn't have to be a formal thing, but it should be a regular thing. It might seem like a strange concept at first. In fact, for the first several months it might feel awkward. But it's important to know where you stand on a regular and ongoing basis. Once you create the routine around checking in, you will discover that your bond is growing tighter, you are more cognizant of each other's needs and how your words and actions affect each other, and you will be more open to have revealing and substantive conversations that solidify you as a partnership as opposed to two individuals in their own worlds who happen to be walking the path together—tempting fate that your paths will diverge and you grow apart.

NIGHTLY THANK-YOUS

Sometimes we forget to let our partner know how much we appreciate him. We assume that he knows. But, more often than not, he doesn't. He doesn't know how much it truly means to you when he spots and buys a red velvet cupcake for you while doing a quick grocery store run. He doesn't fully realize that the afternoon text he sent you right before going into that big meeting gave you an injection of confidence to shine even brighter and nail the sales pitch, landing you the job! He doesn't see how taken care of you feel when he orders for you at the restaurant and remembers that you like your dressing on the side. It's those little things, the teeny tiny unnecessary extras that he does for you throughout the day that show you just how much he is thinking about you. Acknowledge him for it. The more you reward him—with positive reinforcement—for good behavior, the more he will continue to do for you.

What's interesting, though, is that you might not really know how much effort he puts into the relationship on a daily basis. You might not realize how many little things he does to serve, honor, impress, and show that he is thinking about you. You might be too caught up in your world—or worse, taking those little "nothings" for granted. Just as stopping to smell the roses will help you appreciate the simple beauty that is all around you in the world, stopping to notice and acknowledge the effort that your guy puts into your relationship will deepen your appreciation for him.

Or is it vice versa? Are you the one who isn't appreciated for the many little things that you do throughout the day for your guy? Do you feel like you're constantly making an effort, but it's going unnoticed? That is all about to change—tonight.

It's time to establish a new, healthy habit. Like the monthly check-ins, this could feel awkward at first, but each night as you lie in bed together, before you drift into sleep, tell each other the things that you did for each other that made you feel special. It could be as simple as "thank you for putting toothpaste on my toothbrush this morning before I made it into the bathroom" or "thank you for emptying the dishwasher while I was busy on the phone with my mom" or "thank you for telling me that I looked beautiful in my new suit." The first few nights might be a challenge, as you wrack your brain for what he did that made you feel appreciated, seen, special, and loved. But, after a few days, you will start to mentally take notes each time he does those little things. What you also will likely find is that you start to appreciate each other more and you start to want to do more for each other. Do the little things for him, and appreciate the little things he does for you, and your relationship can't help but improve.

CHAPTER 6

When to Call It Quits and Get Over Him

I MISS YOUR SMILE, BUT I MISS MINE MORE: WHEN TO END IT

Those fantasies are never going to be fulfilled. You didn't fail. It just didn't work and it's time to end it. How do you know when a breakup is something you must do? When do you decide that you love him but you love yourself more? Any woman who has ever had a breakup will tell you that she knew. You know when you are making excuses and settling for less than you deserve. You finally get to a place where you know that you have to do it. One of the markers is, "I miss your smile, but I miss mine more." It's time to honor your intuition and not push your relationship to the place where you are being damaged or damaging him.

SIGNS THAT IT'S OVER

- You stop wanting to be your best self.
- You stop putting energy into your appearance (i.e., shaving, make-up) not because you feel comfortable but because you don't care.
- You are making excuses for him.
- You feel like you are settling for less than you deserve.
- You don't want to touch him.
- You make excuses as to why you can't have sex, or even kiss, right now.
- Everything and everyone else is more important than spending time with him.

HOW TO BREAK UP

Is it okay to break up over text? How about e-mail, phone, in person, changing your relationship status on Facebook? Surprisingly, all *but* changing your Facebook status (don't publicly end it until you privately end it) are fine, depending on the timing and a few specific circumstances.

Still, whether you have been out on three dates or living together for three years, no matter how you cut it, breaking up is hard to do. You don't want to hurt him, because he didn't hurt you. You're just not into him, you're bored, you grew apart, you have different goals, you don't have the time, you don't have chemistry, you feel more like friends, you found someone else, you're too different, too the same, you're still not over your ex, you aren't ready for that level of commitment, you want more out of the relationship, your needs aren't being met, it's just not right, you know that he's not the one, you need more or different, he's such a great guy but he's just not great for you, etc. Fact is, you know it's time to end it, you don't want to drag it out any longer, but you have no idea how to do it. Thankfully I do. Here's how.

TEXT

Yes, cutting the line over text is fine if

You have only been out on one to five dates, you are super casual, you haven't had sex, and you aren't "officially" boyfriend and girlfriend. Why did I include all of those qualifiers? Because, especially if you prequalified, it is possible to ascend to a higher, more connected relationship level even after just one to five dates. But if you didn't, a text exit is totally okay. I know, it seems cold, but let's be realistic here: if you're an active dater, you are going out with lots of different guys who just aren't a fit for you. You don't have to make a whole drama around saying that—we're not a fit. Reverse it: if you went out with a guy a couple of times and you liked him but then he called you and said, "Hey Laurel, just want to let you know that I'm just not that into you," you'd feel awful, not to mention awkward!

So what do you say? A simple text saying the following is just fine:

Hey John, I've really enjoyed getting to know you. Thank you for turning me on to Korean food—I never knew how much I liked it! But I just don't feel like we are a romantic fit. I'm sorry, but I truly hope you find an amazing woman.

Or

Thanks for the date last night, Anthony. You're such a genuinely great guy, I just feel like we are in different places right now, and I don't think it makes sense to continue to see each other. I'm so sorry.

Here are other situations in which a text breakup is acceptable:

He's clearly avoiding you. You have called, e-mailed, texted, and even checked up on him on Facebook, Instagram, and Twitter (so you know he's alive), and he still won't respond to you. He's avoidant for some reason and would probably rather you end it over text anyway.

You're in a digital relationship. Sounds weird, I know, but it's fairly common in this day and digital age to have a relationship primarily (or even entirely) over text and maybe Skype. If that's the case, there's no reason to shake up your mode of comfortable communication and out of the blue call him to end it. Just text him.

E-MAIL

E-mail is an excellent way to end it if

You have been dating for up to six months, you're not living together, and you have yet to utter the words "I love you." Again with the qualifying details that are canceled out if you have been in an accelerated relationship within which you have seen each other several times a week, getting raw and deep from the onset and you are connected on a heart level. E-mail is perfect for this type of relationship ending because you have the opportunity to explain yourself without being sidetracked, improperly expressing yourself and coming across the wrong way, losing your nerve and prolonging the inevitable because you "just can't say it," risking him getting defensive and arguing why you're wrong or why it doesn't make sense, and the list goes on and on. Plus, reverse it: if you were dating a guy, you liked him but you weren't super serious, and he called to tell you that you're great, but . . . you would want to hang up and hide! It doesn't feel good to be told that he's not into you—whether on the phone or in person. And the fact is that once the words "it's not working" are said, you really aren't listening anymore anyway. You don't hear him tell you how great you are. All you hear is "It's over; you're not good enough for me." You may try to fruitlessly argue why he shouldn't end it (which can come across as pathetic), or get defensive and bitchy (officially leaving an awful taste in his mouth). E-mail is the way to go.

So what do you say? How you feel, in an honest and vulnerable way. This is not the time to lie or even avoid the truth. Let him know how you feel, without being a cold bitch. He's a good guy, he did nothing "wrong"—you're just not into him. He definitely doesn't deserve a mean, hasty, blaming, or totally avoidant brush-off just because you're scared, embarrassed, over it, or you feel bad. Instead, you want to tell him how much you have enjoyed spending time with him. Tell him what's happening in your mind and why it's not working for you in a clear and concise way. The e-mail shouldn't be of novel length, but it also shouldn't be just a sentence. If you're open to it, end the e-mail saying that you are happy to talk to him about it over the phone if he wants to talk.

If you're in one of these less common but still relevant situations, an e-mail is also acceptable.

You're in a long-term digital relationship consisting of texts, Skype, and e-mail as your primary methods of connection, so keep up the physical distance and end it over e-mail.

You are unable to connect in any other way because of distance, time, or disconnection. Just because you can't talk on the phone or see each other in person doesn't mean you can't end it. The last thing you want to do is stay in it because you don't want to do an e-mail breakup and then cheat because you're over it in your mind anyway. Not okay.

He's a real asshole. He cheated, lied, stole, manipulated, conned, or hurt you. Instead of having to endure an ugly phone call or in-person conversation, tell him exactly how you feel over e-mail. Or simply say, "It's over. What you did was unacceptable and unforgivable. Do not ever contact me again. I don't want to hear your excuse."

He's dangerous. If it's a safety issue, I don't care how long you have been together, you don't owe him anything. Send him a curt e-mail, then block him and cut him out of all areas of your life.

PHONE

No matter how sure you are that breaking up is what you need to do, actually speaking that truth is a painful call. Not just for him but for you, too. So when do you phone in your breakup?

You have been dating for up to six months, you're not living together, and you have yet to utter the words "I love you." Yup, just like the e-mail breakup when it comes to qualifiers, but the phone breakup is a slightly more personal (and potentially more awkward) mode of breakup communication. It's best to have a script or at least talking points prepared for this phone call to ensure that you stay on track with your purpose, keep it brief but honest, and not chicken out just because you get nervous or feel bad or he gets defensive. To increase your chances of getting your points out in an authentic but kind way, avoid the small talk. Go right into the reason you are calling (to break up), explain why, and finally say that you are sorry but you truly do wish him the best. Don't say "good luck." It sounds bitchy.

You are physically apart. Just because you're physically apart and a face-to-face breakup is impossible doesn't mean that you can't end it. Whether it's a long-distance relationship or you are in different cities for short-term circumstances, the phone breakup is completely acceptable.

IN PERSON

This is a hard conversation to have no matter how over it you both are. If you are in a serious relationship, you live together, you're engaged, married, or "engaged to be engaged," an in-person breakup is the only way to go. You owe it to him to be honest, vulnerable, emotional, and present. It's less about looking at each other in the eye and more about giving the relationship and each other the respect that you deserve after all of this time and after the love that you shared, even if it's ending. If it helps, write a letter and read it. You can also bring talking points to make sure you stay on track. If he comments that it's lame to bring talking points, tell him that you just want to make sure that you honestly express your feelings instead of getting caught up in emotion. Be sweet to him. Don't start an unnecessary fight. If it helps, you can make him feel like it's his idea. I'm not suggesting that you be manipulative or play games, but if you allow him to see your side and see why he would benefit from being apart, he just might come to the same conclusion that you already have. Once you finish the conversation, hug (don't kiss), wish each other well, and say good-bye. You will miss him. You will want to text him to check in. You will want him to share in your daily ups and downs. You will miss having him there as your friend. But don't let that attachment to his comfort and friendship allow you to go back into something that you *know* isn't enough for you.

NOW WHAT?

None of this "Let's finalize the breakup in person" bullshit. If you broke up in any way besides in person, and he wants to finalize it face-to-face, that's a swift no. Um . . . hello breakup sex! And definitely don't go out to dinner for a final good-bye. Why? Because now that you don't have the relationship pressure and there isn't as much weight on what he says, does, or doesn't do or say, you very likely will get along better than you have in a long time . . . which could lead to you suddenly "forgetting" why you broke up in the first place, getting back together, and re-entering the relationship make up / break up cycle. If you want to get back with your ex some time down the line, that's another discussion. But for now, while everything is fresh, cut the line completely.

"Let's meet so we can exchange our stuff." This is a tough one because if you spent much time at his place, or he at yours, there is a high likelihood that some of your stuff currently resides there, and, let's face it, you really do want it back. Still, an in-person stuff exchange is yet another excuse to get together and hash it out—in bed. If jumping in bed is truly off the table, this stuff exchange has the potential to be seriously awkward, filled with anger, or simply depressing, which can again lead to giving it another shot, as discussed above. So here's what you do: either (a) meet at a public place like a park where you can pull your cars next to each other and transfer your stuff, then have a nice hug good-bye, or (b) drop off the stuff outside each other's doors when you know that the other person isn't home. This way you avoid the uncomfortable interaction, and you still get your stuff back.

"I love you . . . but we simply aren't a fit." Your breakup was as friendly as it could possibly be. You parted ways saying "I love you" and knowing that you truly do want to see each other happy in other relationships. Regardless, you have to take a break and completely disconnect for at least several months. Why? You need to break the bond and make room for someone else to come into your life. As comfy as he is to snuggle with and watch TV, that's not his role anymore. As much as you want to call him and let him know what crazy thing your bitch boss did this week, that's not his role anymore. As connected as he was with your dog and as much as you know he will really appreciate knowing that she finally got over her fear of the ocean and followed you into the surf, that's not his role anymore. Don't believe me? Reverse the roles. What if you started dating a guy who was seriously *just* friends but really, *really* close friends with his ex-girlfriend. When they hung out together, you could see that familiar glint in their eyes. Whenever something, anything, happened in your man's life, he made sure to call his ex to share it with her first because she'll find it funny or because she will get it or because she knows the person he's talking about . . . feels shitty, doesn't it? If you have an old but comfy car parked in the garage (and it's just a one-car garage), there is no room to park a new one. Get rid of the old car so that you can make room for the new one. No contact. "I love you, I'll miss you, but we can't communicate for a while." Now take a break.

Take a break. You love each other. You have chemistry. You have fun together. He's a great guy. He gets you and you get him. There is a comfort there. But you or he, simply and sadly, just aren't in the place you need to be in your life in order to make this relationship last . . . right now. That doesn't mean that you won't be in the right place in the future. But you know that if you keep moving forward as a couple at this time, you will end up resenting each other because you are at two different places right now. The question is: can you do the work that you need to do in order to ascend as an individual—together? Or do you need to take a break, work on yourself, and see if you are still a fit later?

WHEN YOU HAVE NO CHOICE
BUT TO BREAK YOUR OWN HEART

Love is easy. But that doesn't mean it's healthy or meant to be. Never will be. No matter how deeply you love the guy—to the depths of your soul, with each breath you take, if you could drink him you would, he is like a drug. You crave him but he's killing you. You're in a bad relationship. And that's when it's time to break up. Breaking your own heart can be the most torturous and confusing breakup of all, because you can't help but question whether you're making the right move. You know you're unhappy, you aren't getting what you need in the relationship, but your heart feels like it is splitting in two, even though you're the one ending it.

Being in a bad relationship can lead to depression, a lifetime of insecurities, unhealthy behaviors and thoughts, and a temporary loss of self. It's time to walk away. Run if you think it's necessary. Eventually your love will fade, and you'll stop thinking about him every minute. Then one day you'll realize that you didn't think about him for days. And in time he fades away....

HOW DO YOU KNOW YOU'RE
IN A BAD RELATIONSHIP?

- He is physically or emotionally abusive.

- You don't like who you are when you're with him.

- You feel like you're suffocating.

- You are lonelier when you're with him than you are when you're alone.

- He is possessive of you in an unhealthy way.

- He doesn't celebrate your accomplishments but would rather one-up you instead.

- He puts you down when you're with other people and makes you feel like an idiot.

- You're afraid that he will get mad at you when you talk to or hang out with your friends, so you feel like you have to lie.

- He checks your phone because he is convinced that you are cheating—but you aren't.

- You can't remember the last time you smiled.

It's time to end it. The sooner you do, the sooner you will smile again. I promise you. It's a little like exercising when you so don't want to. One more day of exercising is one less day of being overweight, is one day closer to reaching your goal.

The same situation applies with breakups: one less day of being together is one day closer to being happy.

EIGHT STEPS TO STOP OBSESSING OVER HIM

Whether the relationship was good or bad, we still tend to be seriously bummed about it when it's over, and we have a really hard time getting over it. *Even* if the relationship was honestly awful, we still struggle to stop thinking about him, oddly "forgetting" all of the bad stuff and just remembering the good. No more saturating in your misery! Instead of sitting there stringing together the moments of good in your mind, do these eight things to stop obsessing and get over him!

Block him on Facebook so he can't check your wall. But more than that, so you can't check his. Social media is one of the worst things when it comes to getting over an ex, as it encourages connection from a distance. You don't want the temptation, nor do you want him to be tempted to reach out.

Stop following him on Twitter and Instagram. He likely will be targeting some tweets and pics toward you, giving you little jabs by showing off other girls, mentioning some of your favorite things, or discreetly inviting you over by posting a photo of your favorite bottle of wine, paired cheese, and "Waiting for you to come and enjoy them with me . . . " just to see if you will take the bait.

Write down the bad. It's too easy to fantasize about the good old days, the things that he was great at, the amazing moments that you shared, and forget about all the bad that you endured and the less than awesome way he treated you. It's time to remind yourself! Write down a list of reasons you broke up in the first place. Each time you start wistfully remembering the good, pull out the sheet of paper covered in the bad and be proud of yourself for sticking to your guns and staying true to you.

Stop crying and start dating! It's not about getting into another relationship; it's not even necessarily about going out on dates; it's about window-shopping your future options and seeing that, yes, there really are lots of fish in the sea. And you know what? Many of them are much better than your ex! So, late at night when you are feeling lonely and sad, instead of fixating on your relationship, stalking your ex on social media, flipping through old photos and letters, or worse—texting or calling him (!)—go online and get an eyeful of some eye candy.

Refresh your look. This doesn't mean chop off your bra strap-length hair to a bob or dye it from golden blonde to dark brown. This means to get a few highlights, a sassy new lipstick, and even a fab pair of stilettos that make you feel oh so sexy!

Have a fabulous girl's night in! Get dolled up, serve champagne cocktails, and have fun again!

Reconnect with yourself. Breakups are all about bummers with benefits! Extract the good from the bad. Think about what lessons you learned, how you have changed, and what you will do differently next time.

Explore your passions. Join a meet-up and go on hikes with a bunch of like-minded locals. Sign up for a cooking class and learn how to make Spanish tapas. Buy a one-month yoga class pass (if you buy in bulk, you are more likely to go). You have time to spare, so spend it well by working on yourself.

UNHOOKING:
ENDING A TOXIC RELATIONSHIP WITH AN EX

I could actually imagine hundreds of hooks in my heart, each with a line at the end pulling in different directions. And at the end of every line was him. He was like a fisherman or a puppeteer, controlling me with every word over text, tone in his voice on the phone, or simply his presence that seemed to linger in everything and almost everyone. I wanted to move on. I craved being in a healthy, loving relationship. But more than that, I wanted to be in a healthy and loving relationship with him. As badly as I knew I needed to unhook him from my heart, I wasn't ready to feel the ache of emptiness without him. I was addicted.

The only cure to an addiction is removing yourself from the situation, detoxing, and coming to grips with the fact that you can never reach out. You have to force yourself not to cyberstalk, ask around about him, or do a drive-by in hopes of catching a glimpse of him or even just his car parked on the street. And you just have to accept the fact that you might not feel that way again in your next relationship, and that's okay. You might not need him; every time you see him you probably won't want to literally swallow him up as your body grows numb from complete chemical bliss. But you will be healthy and happy, you will be the priority, and you will have a balanced life, and that's better than this, right? Right? . . . Yes, that's right.

We had been together, on and off, for years. Years of yo-yoing. Years of extreme passion—both good and bad. Years of repeating the same mistakes. I felt like I was on one of those amusement park rides where you are pinned to a wall that is spinning so fast, then the floor drops out and you are still frozen in place. Then one day I was hit with a shocking realization: I wasn't actually backed up against a wall at all. I was backed up against self-doubt, bad habits, and old obsessions. All I had to do was turn around and start fresh.

When I decided that I couldn't and wouldn't ever go back again, I wailed in a way that I didn't know I had the capacity to sound. I collapsed on the carpet and sobbed for days. I couldn't eat, couldn't exercise because I was too weak, and couldn't work. I wanted to call him, even just so we could fight, because I had come to find comfort in "fuck you, I hate you" phone and text conversations—just feeling connected to him had felt good. Without that connection, I felt purposeless and pathetic. My body didn't take it well. My mind had lost all hope and purpose. I lacked any and all motivation except to feed the dog and open the door to let her out. I shut off my ringer so I wouldn't be bothered by my concerned family and their repeated attempts to check in on me and make sure I was still alive, and I succumbed to the sofa to cry for days. Honestly, I felt like there wasn't a point anymore. Why go on? I felt truly and completely empty. All I could hear were the nasty things he had said to me—"You have no idea how to love and you don't deserve to be loved," "You are the most selfish and disgusting person I have ever known," "Your dog deserves better than you," "You are worthless. . . . "

I needed a new perspective and a change of scenery. I needed to see that there was no wall behind me; it was just me against me. If only I could turn around, I would see. And so I did. I changed my mind, and eventually my heart and life followed. But it took time, sometimes agonizing time. The key was to remove myself from the triggers that flooded my life. I had to create new habits, distance myself from certain friends, find a new hiking trail for my daily workout. I even moved to a different area because I knew that the place I lived was saturated with unavoidable triggers. The only way that I could get away from him was to get away from all that reminded me of him. I wasn't running away. I was hitting the reset button and starting fresh.

* * *

Toxic relationships can be completely debilitating. More than shitty relationships, they can derail your career, force a wedge between you and your friends, and completely destroy your self-worth (what you deserve), sense of self (who you are), and self-sufficiency (your ability to take care of yourself). You may have convinced yourself (possibly with his brainwashing help) that it's really not that bad. He doesn't hit you or anything. He doesn't call you a c**t, bitch, or whore—or maybe he does. He can be very loving to you, sometimes. So let me ask you: Why do you often feel that awful, alone, insecure, scared, worthless, stupid, or small? Healthy relationships don't make you feel that way.

But you know this because you ended it with your now-ex. You got yourself out of that toxic relationship because you knew it wasn't serving you. In fact, it was hurting you. Your wings felt clipped. Your ego was non-existent. You were almost a different person when you were with him, as if you had two personalities: the strong, fun one your friends and family saw, and the half person your guy cut you down to be. Or did you lose yourself completely?

And now you are alone and missing the comfort of him. It's so easy to forget about the bad moments, isn't it? You romanticize the relationship, allowing your mind to wander into the moments—which are truly moments—when you were great. But let's be honest, bad or good, you miss him. So you text a photo of something that reminds you of him. Or you write down the lyrics to a song about heartbreak and e-mail it to him. You stalk him on social media and the feelings come washing over you like a tidal wave. You can't stop obsessing. Sure, he told you that you were worthless, but he also told you that he never loved anyone like he loved you. And you remember when he treated you in that loving way—way back in the day. And he somehow convinces you that if you are "well behaved" and you don't piss him off, he'll go back to being that guy . . . so you go back to him. And soon you fall into a new cycle—the break up / get back together cycle. You stay until you can't stand it anymore, so you leave. But then you miss him unbearably, so you go back.

Let me tell you right now—things won't change. You are addicted. Just like a drug, you are addicted to an unhealthy thing that gives you massive highs and destructive lows. It's the roller coaster that fuels you. You mistake that intense passion for intense love. But you're wrong. You are spiraling in a cycle that you won't be able to pull him out of. You have to be the one to make the decision to step out of it and move on. It's a decision you have to make. And it's not an easy one. But if you want to find true and real love, you have no other choice. Once you make the decision, you have to take the steps to follow through. That means removing yourself from the triggers that tempt you to go back.

Once you make the decision, go back to page 1 of this book. Reset, rebuild, and find love in yourself first, then you *will* find someone better and more amazing for you. The harder you slam a ball into the ground, the higher it bounces back up. A divorce, a breakup, losing a job, or just feeling seriously down can ground you, rough you up a bit, and leave calluses on your feet and grit under your fingernails. But, more than that, it leaves you wiser and stronger next time. Life is about experiencing opposites, isn't it?

CHAPTER 7

You Can Have It All

In many ways I was reading my own script. I had designed a strategy to get guys to fall in love fast. I had an ideal in my mind of what type of guy made the most sense for me—he was super successful, emotionally strong, confident to the edge of cocky, quirky, crazy about me, dynamic, interesting, and wanted a serious relationship that would soon lead to a family. Because my strategy works—almost too well—it was easy to find, reel in, catch, and keep almost any guy I wanted. I said and did the right things, set up the perfect emotional environment that would make him (lots of hims) fall deep, hard, and fast for me, and I was home free. But something was missing—me. I wasn't feeling it.

These were great guys. Almost every one of them. I would rave about them to my family and friends, rattling off their accolades, essential stats, and status that made them worthy of being in a relationship with me, as if I was justifying why we were together. Still, I often felt like I was trying to convince myself that I was crazy about them. Somehow each relationship was crippled by the inability to be "it all":

- He may have been interesting and successful, but I didn't want to have sex with him.

- He may have been emotionally stirring, he may have treated me like a princess, and the sex may have been great, but it was the buildup–kissing, touching, making out–that made me feel like I was being groped . . . until the lights were off and we descended into our emotional depths, beyond the reality of the physicality.

- He may have been comforting and may have created a feeling of home, but somehow I felt unimportant and undervalued when I was with him.

- He may have intellectually thrilled me and the sex may have been chemically addictive, but he was emotionally and verbally insensitive and made it clear that I wasn't a priority.

I rationalized each relationship by repeating to myself two things that had been said to me—"When is enough, enough?" and "Life isn't a fairytale and you won't find a prince. No one can have it all. And no one includes you." So I would tell myself, "Laurel, he's successful, he's crazy about you, he's nice to you . . . What's wrong with that?" or "Laurel, you have great sex, he pushes you intellectually, you're proud to be with him, what could be better?" or "Laurel, he's comforting and makes you feel at home, why do you need more than that?" And I almost had myself convinced. It's not that I was settling per se, but I made the decision that enough was enough.

Don't get me wrong; it's not that I was acting when I was around them. When we were together I was fully present and engaged. It's just that I preferred to be alone. I had other priorities. And that felt perfectly acceptable. My days were packed full with work obligations—which always came first. After giving so much of myself to my work, I had little left to give to them.

Because I was offering crumbs, they would become needy and ask for more, making me feel like I was suffocating as their sad and rejected eyes would drop each time I wouldn't sleep over, was too focused on work to have a clear enough mind for sex, or couldn't find the time to see them again that week . . . Which made me feel even more smothered. Sick of always being the leaver, sometimes I would make myself completely inaccessible while seeding the idea in their minds that they would be better off if we weren't together, so that they would end it with me. And the cycle began again as I put my strategy into practice with another fantastic man . . . Who turned out to somehow not be quite right either. Feeling like the princess and the pea, I decided to stop the cycle and, like musical chairs, sit in the next seat that I landed in front of. And I was happy enough. I would get used to the sex. Maybe the chemistry would come. And, anyway, chemistry fades.

And then I went to a party where I overheard a woman talking about her husband and how they had the most intense chemistry, he stimulated her emotionally and intellectually, she felt like the luckiest woman every day, and next week was their twenty-year anniversary. I was jealous.

Two weeks later, I met him. He wasn't super business- and money-driven. He was tall, dark, and handsome. He was younger. Three things that would historically be an instant turnoff for me. But there was something about him that I couldn't get enough of. And it wasn't just the sex, the taste of his skin, the smell of him that lingered even after he left. It wasn't that his intense masculinity made me feel incredibly feminine and sexy. It wasn't that we couldn't watch TV together because we would end up talking over and pausing the show so often that it would take five hours to get through a one-hour episode. It wasn't that I felt like a giddy schoolgirl around him. It wasn't that he made me feel comfortable to be my authentic self for the first time in more than ten years. It wasn't that he was the breath beneath my wings, always encouraging me to be my best self. It wasn't that I was proud to enter a room with him, knowing how many eyes were fixated on his strapping good looks. It wasn't that he never annoyed me. It wasn't that I loved snuggling with him (which I had decided years before just wasn't me—I wasn't the snuggling type). It wasn't that I actually enjoyed having him sleep over (which I had previously never been comfortable with). It was all of it combined. As soon as we met, my priorities and perspective shifted, and work was no longer the center of my world. I woke up and fell asleep smiling. I found myself introducing him as "this is my boyfriend, and he makes me so happy," instead of "this is my boyfriend and this is what he does for a living, and he lives in this amazing neighborhood and last weekend he took me on vacation to this amazing place." I no longer felt the need to justify why I chose him by talking up his wealth and status. He made me happy. And that was what mattered.

And that's when I realized that you *can* have it all. "It all" just might look different than what you had in mind.

But remember: All rules are meant to be broken.

ACKNOWLEDGMENTS

To my clients: the amazing women who inspire me every day to continue being my best self, so that I can help you be your best selves too.

Steve. I have never in my life felt so loved, so adored, and so deserving of being a priority. Thank you for loving all my curves and all my many edges. And thank you for allowing me to see myself through your lens.

To the men I have loved, who have loved me, and who left an imprint ... Thank you for the lessons. Thank you for enduring me during my many moments of weakness when I said and did—and didn't say or do—things in ways that were not aligned with my best self. Those experiences helped me to grow and develop into the coach I am today.

Rich. Thank you for being my reality-checking voice of reason and wisdom when mine was lacking. Thank you for always being there for me with my best interests in mind. Thank you for making me smile and exhale and think and introspect. And thank you for the red velvet cupcakes.

Tony. Thank you for being my forever friend since childhood, allowing me to make mistakes without judgment and knowing, accepting, and loving the real me always.

Marni. Thank you for giving me the opportunity to work with such amazing women—you included. You are an inspiration.

Christine. I have always been awed by your beauty, strength, grace, and all-knowingness.

Alisa. You are truly the only one who has been there and seen all of it. You have supported my crazy "only happens to Laurel" adventures with men and helped me see the reality through the fantasy. Thank you for being a sounding board, allowing me to get real and deep, and being a source of levity.

Bekah. Thank you for your tenderness and friendship. Thank you for allowing me to let my guard down with you and, as you said, be human.

Deb. Thank you for the eight-mile love, life, and work intensives. Thank you for getting me out of my box and into the real world for a breath of fresh air and a muscle-burning workout.

Roger Chatten. Thank you for reminding me when I had momentarily lost me.

Anthony Mattero. Thank you for believing so completely in me and helping me hone and bring a broader voice to my brand. Your honest and sometimes brutal notes made me so much better.

Cindy De La Hoz. This book would not be if not for you. Thank you for letting me be my authentic self, encouraging my true voice, and not editing out my edge.

Mom, Dad, Julia, Garth. Thank you for enduring my screwing-the-rules attitude throughout my life. Julia, thank you for inspiring me to teach my lessons . . . so that you don't make my many mistakes. Garth, thank you for getting me and truly being there for me, even when I wasn't there for myself. Dad, thank you for challenging me with "When is enough, enough?" Mom, thank you for reminding me "Enough of the lessons, Laurel . . . it's time to live."

XX Laurel